Working with

Dysphagia

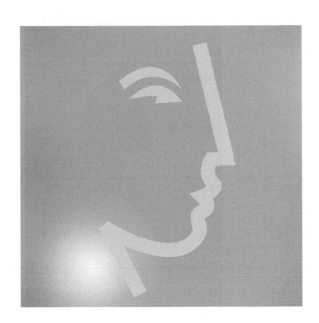

Lizzy Marks
& Dierdre Rainbow

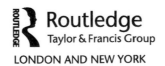

Routledge
Taylor & Francis Group

LONDON AND NEW YORK

DEDICATION

To Adrianne Marks, who kindled and supported her daughter Lizzy's interest and enthusiasm for working as a speech and language therapist, and to all our colleagues, clients, their families and carers, from whom we have learnt so much.

First published 2001 by Speechmark Publishing Ltd.

Published 2017 by Routledge
2 Park Square, Milton Park, Abingdon, Oxon OX14 4RN
711 Third Avenue, New York, NY 10017, USA

Routledge is an imprint of the Taylor & Francis Group, an informa business

British Library Cataloguing in Publication Data

Marks, Lizzy
  Working with Dysphagia
  1. Deglutition disorders – Treatment   2. Speech therapy
  I. Title   II. Rainbow, Deirdre
  616.3'1'06

ISBN: 9780863882494 (pbk)

Contents

Figures

TABLES

Acknowledgements

We should like to offer our grateful thanks to the following colleagues for their generous help and time: Diana Moir, Gillian Kennedy, Sara Dibben, Adrianne Marks, Clare Foster, Amanda Hill, Justine Slattery, Liz Clark, Sue McGowan, Fiona MacMahon, Theo Read, Alyson Warland, Liz Knapp, Russell Don, Helena Gibson, Sharon Croxford, Alexa Scott, Lian Soo, Sheila Hayles, Jackie Murray-Leonard, Gary Maughn, Peter Marsden, Dr John Goldstone, Dr Janice Fiske, Karen Hyland, Kirsten Turner, and all the staff, clients and their families of University College London Hospitals, St Pancras Hospital and Camden and Islington Community Health Services NHS Trust.

We should like to express our appreciation to Judith Langley, for her contribution in the form of her original book, *Working with Swallowing Disorders*, which has shaped and influenced us as clinicians.

Finally, our special thanks to our husbands, Jonathan Weinreich and Paul Richmond, and to Stephanie Martin, for their constant encouragement and support, without whom this book would not have been possible.

Foreword

Within recent years there has been a marked increase in the number of referrals to speech and language therapy departments of patients presenting with swallowing problems. Not only has this endangered debate within the profession itself regarding the subsequent impact on the level of services provided to communicatively impaired clients, but it has created further demand on already stretched resources.

Nevertheless, it is wholly appropriate for speech and language therapists to have become an integral part of the multidisciplinary team working with patients presenting with dysphagia. Their knowledge and skills base gives the speech and language therapist unique understanding both of the swallow process and the communicative and sociological issues that are affected when eating and drinking abilities are impaired through neurological insult.

Accompanying the growth of work in the area of dysphagia is a concomitant expansion in research and literature with speech and language therapists making significant contributions to these arenas.

Lizzy Marks and Deirdre Rainbow have worked extensively with patients presenting with dysphagia following neurological impairment. This book is based on their own practical experiences of assessing and managing swallowing disordered clients both in acute and non-acute settings. Their writing not only reflects the considerable knowledge each has amassed over the years but shows humility in acknowledging that, no matter how experienced and skilled, the speech and language therapist is only one component of the dysphagia team.

This book will be a useful resource for all therapists, ranging from student to specialist, as the practical assessment approach and comprehensive management strategies are supported throughout with references of recent relevant research.

Gillian Kennedy
Specialist Speech & Language Therapist
University College London Hospital
June 2001

Introduction

'When a person is unable to swallow, the ability to enjoy almost all other aspects of life is affected. Even minor, intermittent dysphagia can lead to psychological and social stresses. Episodes of choking can lead to a fear of eating that can lead to malnutrition and social withdrawal' (McCulloch *et al*, in Perlman & Schulze-Delrieu, 1997). Speech and language therapists play a key role in reducing the impact of the swallowing impairment, disability and handicap.

As stated in *Communicating Quality 2* (RCSLT, 1996), 'Speech and language therapists work within a climate of rapid change in health, education, social services and voluntary sector settings.' Appropriate management of clients with dysphagia in these settings prevents complications as a result of aspiration, compromised nutrition and dehydration. It is also cost effective compared to admission to hospital for treatment of pneumonia (Groher & Crary, 1997). Our role in the care of people with swallowing difficulties 'is increasingly recognised and advances in medical science are leading to more people surviving with multiple, complex diagnoses. These factors are likely to lead to speech and language therapists contributing increasingly to these difficult decisions' (Rice, 1999). In order to fulfil this role and deliver a high quality service, clinicians need to maintain and expand their knowledge base by enhancing their skills following qualification.

In the past decade, since the publication of Judith Langley's *Working with Swallowing Disorders* in 1988, there have been many changes in public policy, shifts in client profile and research developments in the assessment and management of the client with dysphagia. Our goal is to produce a book that is accessible to speech and language therapists new to dysphagia, particularly of a neurogenic origin, as well as being an up-to-date, evidence-based resource for clinicians already working in this area. We hope to achieve this by providing a sound theoretical background, so that clinicians understand the management implications of various aetiologies, while being highly functional and demonstrating best working practices.

The information presented is applicable to a variety of clinical settings, and stresses the importance of a multidisciplinary approach. The contents are based on our clinical experience of both acute and community-based dysphagia management, from working with a range of patient ages and neurological disorders. However, we have chosen not to include working with clients who have undergone head and neck surgery, as this is covered in *Working with Oral Cancer* (Appleton & Machin, 1995). We appreciate that, in the rapidly expanding field of dysphagia assessment and management, knowledge and practice changes, and so aspects of the text may therefore become out-of-date after writing. We have tried to include current research trends that are functional in a variety of clinical settings.

In addition, this textbook may also be used for reference by physiotherapists, dietitians, occupational therapists, nurses and doctors wishing to further develop their understanding of the nature of dysphagia and its management strategies.

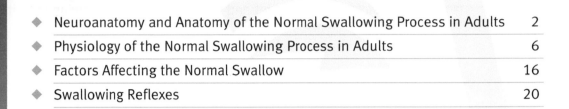

Chapter 1: The Normal Swallow

NEUROANATOMY AND ANATOMY OF THE NORMAL SWALLOWING PROCESS IN ADULTS

This section describes the basic neuroanatomy and anatomy of swallowing. The content has been selected to ensure that the reader can fully comprehend the physiology, assessment and management of swallowing (and its disorders) which follow.

Neuroanatomy

The cranial nerves, seven of which are vital in controlling swallowing, provide both a motor function and sensory information. While they are crucial to the swallowing process, clinicians may experience difficulty in retaining details of their innervation and function. Functional assessments look at the whole swallowing process, rather than individual nerve responses.

In specific cases (such as those resulting from anoxia, or following head and neck surgery) it may be appropriate to look in detail at individual cranial nerves. Therefore, a basic summary of their sensory and motor functions is provided in Table 1.1. The neural control of swallowing is covered later in this chapter.

Anatomical structures

Details of the important anatomical structures are provided in this section. The specific muscles are not detailed, since they are of significance in a functional dysphagia assessment only if one is dealing with a client who has undergone head and neck surgery. This is not the remit of this book. The important anatomical structures are shown in Figure 1.1.

The oral cavity

The oral cavity is separated from the nasal cavity above by an anterior bony hard palate, and a soft (muscular) palate posteriorly. The soft palate is relaxed, allowing an exchange between the two cavities during respiration, but closes during swallowing to prevent nasal regurgitation. The anterior section of the hard palate, directly behind the upper teeth, is known as the alveolar ridge.

Table 1.1 Cranial Nerves and their Function

Cranial Nerve	Sensation	Motor Function
CN I, olfactory	Smell	
CN V, trigeminal	General sensation from the face and muscles of mastication, anterior $\frac{2}{3}$ of tongue	Mandibular movement, elevates soft palate, elevation and anterior movement of larynx
CN VII, facial	Salivation and taste (anterior $\frac{2}{3}$ tongue), soft palate	Muscles of facial expression, elevation of hyoid and tongue base
CN IX, glossopharyngeal	Posterior $\frac{1}{3}$ of tongue, soft palate, faucal arches, mucous membrane of pharynx	Stylopharyngeous muscle
CN X, vagus	Larynx, base of tongue, valleculae and epiglottis, trachea, regulation of depth of respiration and control of blood pressure, nausea	Pharyngeal constrictors, cricopharyngeus, vocal folds
CN XI, accessory		From X via XI: soft palate, pharynx, tongue
CN XII, hypoglossal		Intrinsic and extrinsic tongue muscles, mandible, hyoid and larynx

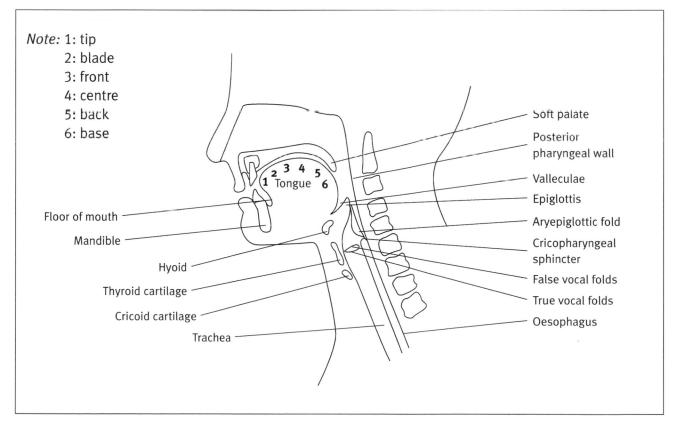

Note: 1: tip
2: blade
3: front
4: centre
5: back
6: base

Figure 1.1 *Lateral view of the head and neck*

The teeth arise from (or dentures attach to) an upper and lower jaw, the maxilla and mandible. The latter is mobile. Externally the jaws are bounded by the cheeks and lips, with the areas between these structures termed the sulci (lateral and anterior).

Within the oral cavity the muscular tongue is the most important structure. The oral section of the tongue includes the tip, blade and back. The body of the tongue sits on the hyoid bone, which is suspended from the oral cavity by the muscles of the floor of the mouth.

There are three pairs of major salivary glands within the oral cavity – the parotids, sublinguals and submandibulars. Further details of saliva production and function are provided in Chapter 6 'Oral Stage Management'. Final important markers in the oral cavity are the anterior faucal arches situated in front of the palatine tonsils (see Figure 1.2). These small areas are considered important in triggering the pharyngeal stage of the swallow.

The larynx

The cartilaginous larynx is suspended from the hyoid bone by the extrinsic laryngeal muscles. Therefore, if the hyoid elevates, the larynx must also rise, unless it is stabilised by musculature within the neck or shoulders. Situated in front of the hypopharynx, the larynx consists of the epiglottis, the thyroid cartilage, the cricoid

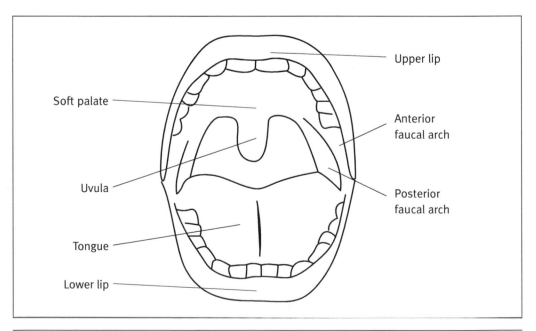

Figure 1.2
Anterior and posterior faucal arches

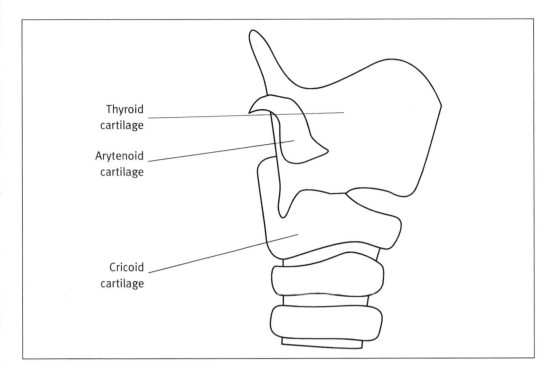

Figure 1.3
The laryngeal cartilages

Thyroid
cartilage

Arytenoid
cartilage

Cricoid
cartilage

cartilage and a number of intrinsic and extrinsic muscles (see Figure 1.3). The trachea is below the larynx.

Of greatest significance in the evaluation of swallowing disorders are (a) the valleculae, the wedge-shaped spaces at the base of the tongue on each side of the epiglottis, and (b) the false vocal folds and the true vocal folds (cords), lying within the thyroid cartilage (see Figure 1.4).

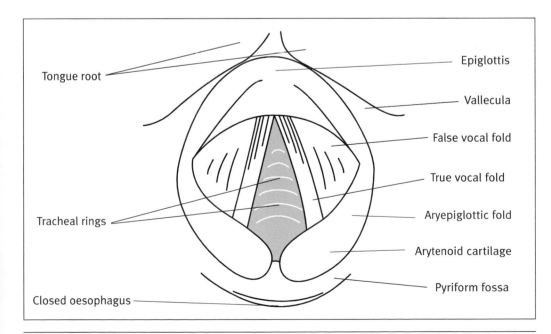

Tongue root

Tracheal rings

Closed oesophagus

Epiglottis

Vallecula

False vocal fold

True vocal fold

Aryepiglottic fold

Arytenoid cartilage

Pyriform fossa

Figure 1.4
Interior of larynx

The pharynx

The pharynx can be divided into three areas: (a) the nasopharynx, which lies above the soft palate, (b) the oropharynx, lying posterior to the oral cavity, and (c) the hypopharynx, or lower portion of the pharynx.

Three muscular constrictors (superior, medial and inferior) form the posterior and lateral walls of the pharynx, attaching to structures situated anteriorly. These anterior bony and soft tissues are the soft palate, the tongue base, the mandible, the hyoid bone, and the thyroid and cricoid cartilages. At the point where the inferior constrictor attaches to the sides of the thyroid cartilage, bilateral spaces known as the pyriform fossae or pyriform sinuses are formed.

Directly below the pyriforms, the pharynx is closed from the oesophagus by the cricopharyngeus muscle (also known as the cricopharyngeus, the upper oesophageal sphincter, the UES, the pharyngo-oesophageal sphincter, cricopharyngeal sphincter or the PE segment).

The oesophagous

Situated behind the trachea, the oesophagus is a collapsed muscular tube, averaging 24cm in length. Closure is maintained by the cricopharyngeal muscle at the top and the lower oesophageal sphincter (or LES) at the bottom.

PHYSIOLOGY OF THE NORMAL SWALLOWING PROCESS IN ADULTS

Speech and swallowing – what is the relationship?

The premise of this book is that there is no relationship between the processes of speech and swallowing, other than shared anatomical structures. Kennedy *et al* (1993) reported, 'In patients with cerebrovascular accidents, swallowing or speech may improve independently of each other (Netsell, 1986). In Parkinson's disease severe dysarthria may exist with minimal or no dysphagia and the reverse (Sarno, 1968; Duvoisin, 1982). These observations are consistent with Netsell's (1986) suggestion that there are specialised and differentiated neurones for speech and swallowing acts .... . Thus, though both behaviours share the same anatomical structures, the actions of each are controlled by different command centres. At a clinical level this suggests that assessing one dysfunction in patients with neurological swallowing and communication difficulties may tell us little of the other.'

The stages of swallowing

The swallowing process consists of four stages: the oral preparatory, oral, pharyngeal and oesophageal. In reality, these stages do not occur in as discrete a way as detailed below; instead, the process is very rapid, with some overlap.

Oral preparatory stage

The level of preparation is dependent on the consistency of the material (known as the bolus) to be swallowed – solid, semi-solid or fluid. Fluid includes saliva. This is a fully voluntary stage, but where does it begin? When one picks up food or a drink, or when the bolus passes the lips? An increasing number of authors (including Leopold & Kagel, 1997) are proposing five stages, including an earlier, pre-oral ingestion stage. Clinical experience indicates that the more one can do to ensure that a person is ready to eat or drink and can participate in the self-feeding process, the more normal the oral preparatory and subsequent stages of swallowing. This point will be discussed further below. Influences on the pre-oral stage include state of hunger and thirst; visual and olfactory information; emotional state; milieu of the meal; societal influences; taste (see Figure 1.5); texture; motor skills, including utensil use; hand-mouth coordination; posture; eating rate. Thus the oral preparatory stage takes a variable amount of time.

Saliva is an essential component of this stage. It performs a number of functions – dental and mucosal protection, maintenance of oral pH, antimicrobial action – but most relevant to preparing the bolus for swallowing is its ability to lubricate and assist with bolus formation. Saliva acts as a solvent for the tastants in food, and as a vehicle for delivering the tastant to the taste buds. At this stage, the basic processing of the food into its constituents commences, including the enzymatic breaking down of carbohydrates.

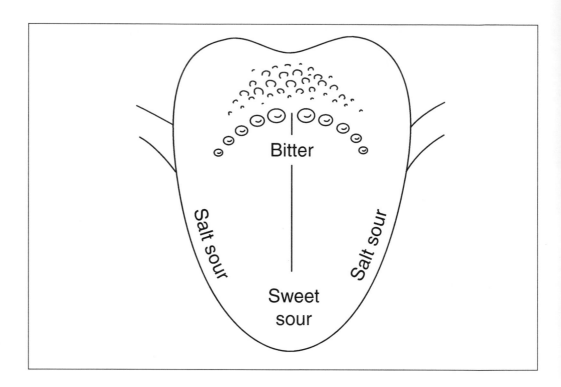

Figure 1.5
Distribution of taste sensors on the tongue

With or without a bolus, insufficient saliva means that a person cannot swallow or execute a dry swallow. Try swallowing consecutively and see how many swallows can be performed without stopping. It is likely that there will be insufficient saliva after three to four swallows and it will be virtually impossible to swallow until the salivary source has been replenished.

Chewing is required to prepare a solid or semi-solid into a bolus that can be swallowed. During this action the food is retained in the oral cavity by lip seal anteriorly. It used to be thought that the bolus was retained posteriorly by contact between the tongue and soft palate, but only intermittent and irregular connection has been observed (Hiiemae & Palmer, 1999). A rotatory jaw movement in a preferred direction grinds the food with saliva to produce a bolus that it is possible to swallow. The food is placed between the molars by a figure-of-eight tongue movement, while the cheek musculature maintains food between the molars and prevents it falling into the sulci.

Oral transit occurs in synchrony with continued food processing, so the bolus is formed and transported while chewing continues. The bolus accumulates on the pharyngeal surface of the tongue and is maintained on that surface without any discernible anatomical constraint. The position of this bolus is constantly changing, although the general trend is descent towards the valleculae. This is normal as long as penetration and/or aspiration do not occur (see below).

With fluids, which have not required earlier preparation, normal healthy adults differ in the rapidity with which they then proceed to the oral stage: some do so immediately; others hold the bolus in this position for a short period prior to swallowing. We suggest the clinician experiments with different types of fluids such as hot, chilled, fizzy and alcoholic drinks, noting the difference between them.

Oral stage

This is the oral transfer stage – the final voluntary section of the swallow. Until recently, texts described this as a discrete stage, which could be initiated only once the oral preparatory stage was complete. However, as mentioned above, Hiiemae and Palmer (1999) recently demonstrated piecemeal oral transit while chewing solid boluses, something that had been difficult to demonstrate because of the limited number of videofluoroscopies performed on normal healthy adults (for safety reasons). This pre-transit movement of the bolus may continue for over 10 seconds, and is highly variable, depending for example on initial consistency of the bolus, age and personal preferences. Thus bolus formation may occur in either the mouth (liquids, very small amounts of food) or the oropharynx (larger volumes of soft and hard foods). Despite this recognition of piecemeal transit, chewing must cease fully, to complete the oral stage.

Wherever the bolus is held, the maximum timescale for this phase is only one second, during which the tongue elevates and rolls posteriorly in a peristaltic motion, sequentially contacting the hard and soft palate. The bolus is moved by lowering the pressure in the mouth which is created by lip and jaw closure, an increase in buccal tone, and anterior and lateral tongue seal against the alveolar ridge. Tongue movement during the oral stage may be described as a stripping action, with the midline of the tongue sequentially squeezing the bolus posteriorly against the hard palate. The sides and tip of the tongue are anchored firmly against the alveolar ridge and upper dentition (or gums in edentulous individuals), forming a central groove or chute. Lip seal is also the norm (and socially acceptable), although not essential, for example, a small number of people may achieve an anterior seal using the upper teeth against the lower lip.

Entry of the bolus into the pharynx coincides with elevation and retraction of the soft palate against the pharyngeal wall, and the onset of the pharyngeal stage.

Pharyngeal stage

The basic life functions of breathing and swallowing rely on two parallel tubes, which occur in close proximity in the human throat: the trachea for respiration, and the pharynx and oesophagus for deglutition. Only one of these functions can occur at any one time. Swallowing requires rapid suspension of respiration and passage of the bolus through the pharynx into the oesophagus, with a resumption of normal breathing after one second. This is the swallow or pharyngeal stage. It is broken down into four sub-stages. The first is elevation and retraction of the soft palate. This action permits the closure of the nasopharynx to avoid nasal regurgitation. The second sub-stage is laryngeal closure and suspension of respiration. Logemann (1998) describes the process of laryngeal closure and opening of the cricopharyngeus as a biomechanical action (see Figure 1.6).

The larynx elevates and tilts forward. This movement pulls the cricopharyngeal muscle, relaxing it to an open position in readiness to receive the bolus (see below). Without this laryngeal movement, the cricopharyngeus cannot open. This movement should be observable and/or palpable (see Figure 1.7).

Elevation of the larynx also enlarges the pharynx to receive the bolus. Next, laryngeal closure and hence suspension of respiration occurs as a result of laryngeal elevation and anterior tilting of the arytenoids, causing them to oppose the base of the epiglottis. Closure takes place at three levels: the true vocal folds, the false vocal folds and the epiglottis covering the larynx as if a lid.

Relaxation and opening of the cricopharyngeus occurs in the third sub-stage. Relaxation precedes opening by approximately one-tenth of a second. Neither

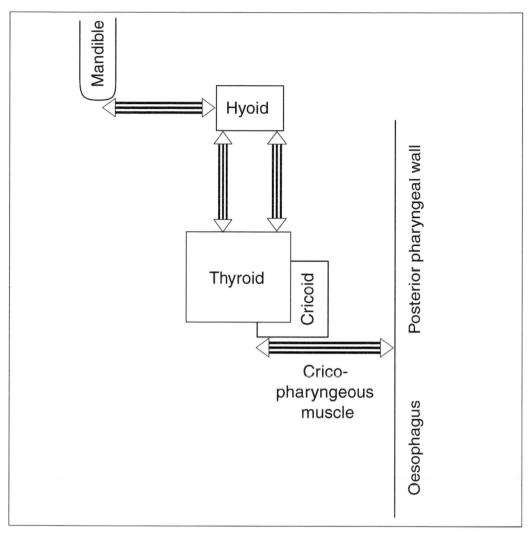

Figure 1.6
Biomechanical opening of the cricopharyngeal muscle

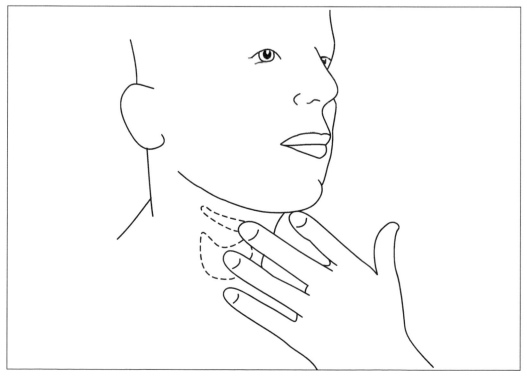

Figure 1.7
Tactile assessment of the swallow

action can be achieved without the laryngeal elevation and tilting detailed above. A bolus entering the pharynx under such circumstances would therefore remain above the cricopharyngeal sphincter, which is normally under tonic closure.

Occasional mistiming of the pharyngeal stage can occur in normal healthy adults, resulting in material entering the airway. The normal response is the triggering of a cough reflex to eject the bolus from a level of penetration (the material penetrates the laryngeal vestibule) or of aspiration (the material penetrates below the level of the vocal folds).

Finally there is bolus propulsion and pharyngeal clearance. It is important both that the bolus is rapidly propelled through the pharynx, given that respiration has been suspended temporarily, and that there is an effective mechanism for clearance of any residue to minimise the risk of penetration or aspiration post-swallow. Two main forces propel the bolus through the pharynx: gravity and base of tongue movement. With a liquid bolus, little other than gravity is required to aid its passage. In addition, the action of the tongue base contacting the posterior wall of the pharynx generates increased intrabolus pressure. This sequential descending contact forces any residue out of the valleculae.

Potential sites of pooling (see Figure 1.8) are the valleculae, the posterior pharyngeal wall and the pyriform fossae. Longitudinal shortening of the pharyngeal constrictors virtually obliterates the laryngeal vestibule and pyriform fossae, avoiding post-swallow residue in these areas. Since this significantly shortens the length of the pharynx, the speed of bolus transit is also increased. In 75 per cent of non-dysphagic adults a liquid bolus splits as it passes through the pyriform fossae (see Figure 1.9), then joins again to pass through the relaxed cricopharyngeus.

Sequential horizontal contraction of the pharyngeal constrictors in a descending pattern, or pharyngeal peristalsis, occurs late in the swallow and appears to be primarily a pharyngeal clearance event rather than part of bolus propulsion.

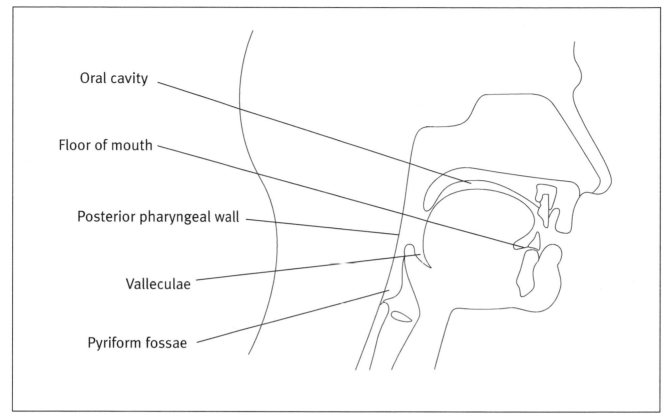

Figure 1.8 *Sites of pooling*

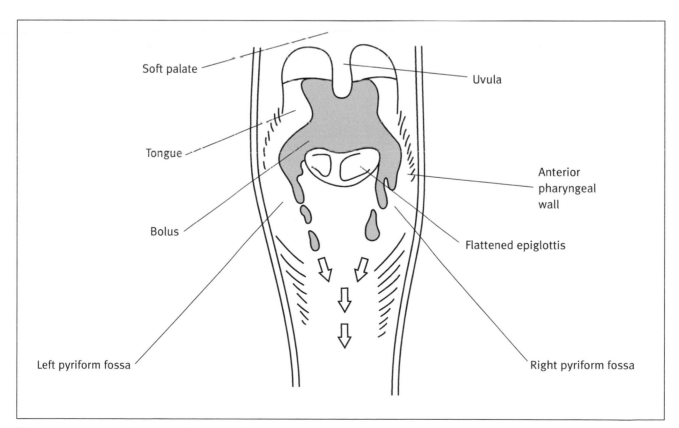

Figure 1.9 *Posterior, anterior view of pyriform fossae: bolus splitting either side of the epiglottis and its pathway through the pyriform fossae*

The base of tongue and pharyngeal constrictors both respond to sensory information to ensure maximal clearance from the valleculae and pyriforms respectively (see 'Neural Control of Swallowing' below). However, swallowing very dry or viscous material may necessitate a second (known as a dry, clearing or check) swallow to clear it fully.

To summarise:

1   The larynx rises and tilts forward, closing at three levels: the true vocal folds, the false vocal folds, with the epiglottis closing over the top. Breathing stops.
2   This movement pulls on the cricopharyngeous muscle at the top of the oesophagus, relaxing it to open.
3   The bolus moves over the back of the tongue, through the pharynx towards the open oesophagus.
4   Bolus transit and clearance are assisted by gravity, the base of the tongue and the pharyngeal constrictors.
5   The bolus enters the oesophagus.
6   Return of the larynx to its normal position. The oesophagus closes, breathing resumes.

Oesophageal stage

The oesophageal stage is under involuntary control. It takes between two and 20 seconds for the bolus to move through the oesophagus by peristaltic action. While this stage is the province of the gastroenterology team, its importance to speech and language therapists working with clients with dysphagia has developed over recent years. Current research suggests that the oesophageal stage affects the oral and pharyngeal stages, since the swallowing system can be viewed as a series of sphincters that create pressure to propel the bolus (see Figure 1.10).

It is virtually impossible to swallow if the oesophagus is full, or emptying very slowly. Dysphagia arising from abnormalities of the oesophagastric region can result in symptoms in the oropharynx and hypopharynx, leading a client to identify the location of the problem higher than the level of the lesion. It is important to remember that problems may coexist at more than one level.

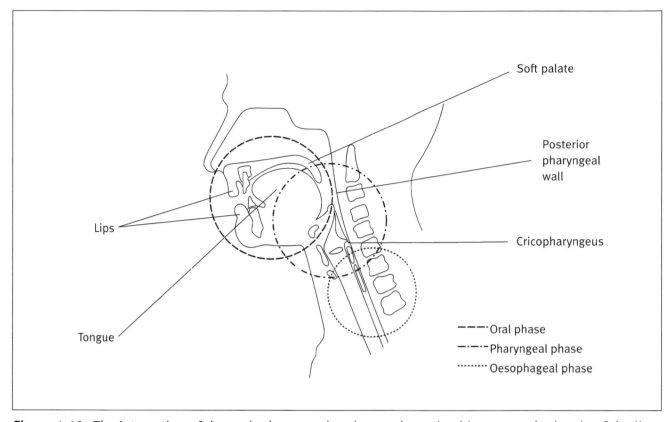

Figure 1.10 *The interaction of the oral, pharyngeal and oesophageal sphincters at the levels of the lips, tongue, soft palate and cricopharyngeus*

Single versus sequential swallows

Single swallows have been widely studied; indeed the physiology of the normal swallow described above has been largely derived from such investigations. But, for most oral intake, single swallows are not the norm. Chi-Fishman and Sonies (1998) described sequential swallows in a small study of normal healthy adults: 'Results revealed that sequential swallows were significantly shorter than discrete swallows in oral transit, pharyngeal response, UES opening, and total swallow durations, but significantly longer in pharyngeal transit and stage transition durations.'

Neural control of swallowing

The oral preparatory and oral stages are described as voluntary, suggesting that they are under cortical control. Evidence is provided by (a) our ability to influence specific movements in the swallowing process, for example deciding to stop chewing, and (b) the use of learned responses, such as keeping your lips closed when chewing because it is socially acceptable.

Hamdy and Power (1998), utilising transcranial magnetic stimulation, indicate that there is a swallowing dominant hemisphere, irrespective of handedness. With regard to recovery after a neurological insult, however, there is evidence that, for some individuals, compensatory reorganisation in the undamaged hemisphere leads to a recovery in swallow function over a period of weeks.

There are two theories regarding how the 'paired swallowing centres', situated in the reticular formation of the medulla, the adjacent sensory or afferent nucleus tractus solitaris, and the motor or efferent nucleus ambiguus, work to produce the swallow (Dodds, 1989). According to the *reflex chain hypothesis*, as the bolus moves through the mouth and pharynx it stimulates sensory receptors that sequentially trigger the next step in the swallow sequence: swallowing proceeds as a chain of linked reflexes each stimulating the next step. The *central pattern generator hypothesis* holds that once swallowing is initiated, it proceeds in a pre-programmed sequence, irrespective of the feedback from the sensory receptors.

The reality is probably a combination of these two theories. Thus there is a central patterned programme laid down for swallowing, which can be modified in line with feedback from the sensory receptors throughout the oral and pharyngeal cavities. Size and consistency of bolus therefore influence the swallow via the reflex chain.

FACTORS AFFECTING THE NORMAL SWALLOW

The theories described above, and particularly evidence for the influence of the reflex chain hypothesis, suggest factors that may affect the normal swallow. Eating and drinking are highly important to most normal healthy adults. Consider how often meals or drinks take place in a social setting. Appetite, food presentation, environment, hygiene (including odours), comfort (including bowels), social situation, mood, and previous life experiences are also influential in eating and drinking.

Detailed below are seven factors that affect the physiology of the swallowing process and that are of considerable importance in the assessment and management of dysphagia.

Posture

Appropriate posture (see Figure 1.11) is fundamental to effective eating and drinking. Besides overall comfort, and permitting gravity to aid the process, there are reasons for ensuring that the swallowing position is ideal. Symmetry and stability promote maximum independence in self-feeding (see below). To achieve this, the relationship of the head to trunk/hip and knee flexion/feet is essential.

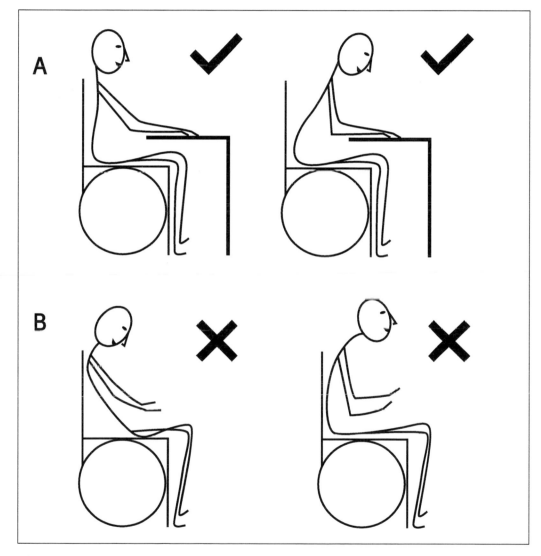

Figure 1.11 *Posture*
(A) Ideal posture involves symmetry: an extended or upright trunk, upright head with chin tuck, flexion at the hips and knees, with both feet flat on the floor.

(B) Unstable posture with curvature of the trunk and without the stable base of the hips and feet.

Figure 1.12
Head flexion to enhance the vallecular space, bringing the epiglottis closer to the pharyngeal wall

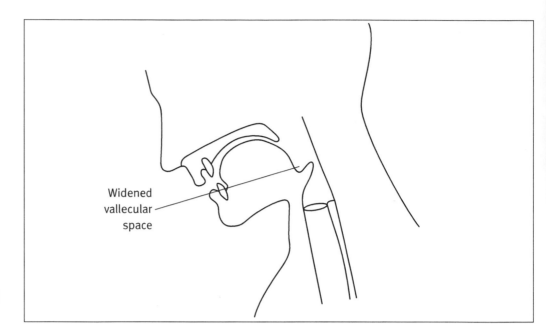

Widened vallecular space

In addition, increased head flexion (see Figure 1.12) increases the vallecular space and brings the tongue closer to the posterior pharyngeal wall (see Chapter 7 'Pharyngeal Stage Management' for rationale).

Self-feeding

The relevance of self-feeding was discussed in the oral preparatory stage above. If fed by another person, one's enjoyment of food and the swallowing process itself may be affected by this loss of control.

Cognitive influences

While cognitive influences may be anticipated following a neurological insult, they are seen in normal healthy adults too. The most common factor is fatigue, resulting in accidents such as biting the inside of the mouth because efferent information is slower. A momentary lapse in concentration (due to fatigue or trying to talk and/or laugh and swallow at once) can result in an embarrassing coughing fit.

Bolus size

Normal healthy adults are able to swallow a large bolus, even when it may be difficult to contain it in the oral cavity when chewing, as it may be swallowed in a piecemeal fashion. Physiologically, a large bolus results in earlier and longer laryngeal closure (and hence airway closure) and longer and wider cricopharyngeus opening.

Bolus viscosity

Research has been carried out using barium, which is naturally very sticky. To reduce the residue from sticky consistencies in the pharynx, the tongue base increases its duration of contact with the posterior pharyngeal wall, in an effort to propel the barium. In parallel, the cricopharyngeus remains open longer to accept the bolus. Videofluoroscopy observations (see Chapter 4) indicate that, in spite of these physiological adaptations, the normal healthy adult may need to engage in multiple dry swallows to fully clear the bolus.

Disuse–dysfunction

Clinicians working with people with voice disorders may be familiar with disuse–dysfunction. For example, the client who has recovered from an episode of laryngitis may remain dysphonic, having lost the normal pattern of phonation. This is usually remedied in one or two voice therapy sessions. A similar situation may be observed with the frailer, older person who becomes unwell, resulting in reduced oral intake, poor nutrition and potential dehydration. They may have little saliva to swallow, which reduces their ability to practise dry swallows to facilitate their swallow function. Once the swallow is re-established, the problem is unlikely to recur.

Normal ageing

Multiple factors have been identified with regard to normal ageing, largely in the 85-year-plus age group. However, it is a problematic area of study as it may be difficult to totally exclude the effects of medication, nutrition and hydration (for example, owing to self-imposed restrictions based on concerns regarding continence).

Fucile *et al* (1998) found that oral stage skills are not age-dependent; instead, good health and natural dentition were more important indicators of preserved functional feeding skills. Yet even those who wore full dentures still performed within the 'normal' range. Three areas commonly noted in clinical assessment of older clients (85 years and over) are the following:

1   Increased number of chews, irrespective of dentition.
2   Reduced pharyngeal peristalsis, resulting in pooling on the pharyngeal wall, necessitating more dry swallows and the use of more moist foods.
3   Reduced oesophageal peristalsis, resulting in increased transit time, hence older people may feel satiated quickly and take longer to complete a meal.

Overall, older people have a reduced reserve capacity that can be recruited as they are, in normal conditions, performing at or near maximum capacity.

SWALLOWING REFLEXES

This section covers the development of normal infant swallowing reflexes and the disappearance of these primitive reflexes to be replaced by normal adult swallowing reflexes. In addition, descriptions of two abnormal reflexes are included. The neurologically impaired client may exhibit primitive and abnormal reflexes. While the latter are never of value, and normally interfere with the swallow, a re-emergence of primitive reflexes may be harnessed to reintroduce oral intake: for example, the use of the rooting reflex to orientate a client to the presence of a spoon.

Reflexes in the newborn

At birth, the infant relies on the fact that it has total reflexive behaviour in order to survive. The oral and pharyngeal reflexes described below have one purpose, that of survival.

Rooting

This is elicited by touching or stroking the cheeks or lips. It causes the infant to turn towards the source of the stimulus, opening the mouth in preparation; its purpose is to locate the source of food. This is how the infant initially finds the breast.

Sucking

Evans Morris and Dunn Klein (1987) describe two distinct phases of the sucking reflex in infant development. The first, suckling, involves a 'definite backward-and-forward movement of the tongue' to draw fluids (or soft food) into the mouth. This develops into sucking, which features a 'raising and lowering of the body of the tongue'. This mature, stronger movement may overlap with the more primitive suckling for some time.

Cough reflex

The cough is a protective laryngeal reflex. In a healthy individual it is generally strong enough to cope with penetration (and occasionally aspiration) of food or fluid, including saliva.

Gag reflex

Like the cough reflex, the gag reflex is also designed for survival. It is the forceful movement of the tongue and reverse peristaltic movement of the pharynx. It serves to prevent ingestion of substances dangerous to swallow, such as solids introduced too early or anything the digestive system cannot cope with, such as poisons, bile or vomit. It can be elicited easily in the child by touching the posterior three-quarters of the tongue or the pharyngeal wall. While the reflex is retained in adults, there is a large range of sensitivity, and it may be partly brought under voluntary control in the fully conscious patient, for example when undergoing a dental or ear, nose and throat examination.

Transverse tongue reflex

The transverse tongue reflex serves only to provide a motor pattern for the lateral tongue movement used in chewing. In infants it can be elicited by touch or taste stimulation applied to the lateral border of the tongue, which then moves towards the stimulus to facilitate bolus formation.

Phasic bite reflex

This is the normal bite and release pattern, elicited by touching the teeth or gums with, for example, a rusk, toy or fingers. It is not a functional bite, but rather a stage in the development of chewing, the repetitive biting rhythm providing an initial experience with a stronger jaw force and the release that follows. By age nine months the infant can hold a rusk between the gums or teeth; the jaw is stabilised in a closed position as the rusk breaks, and the infant chews and swallows the portion in its mouth.

The abnormal reflexes

Tonic bite reflex

All bite reflexes are not the same. A tonic bite reflex can be identified when the infant or adult with neurological damage does not release the bite easily, or when there is tension associated with it. It interferes with all aspects of feeding. Elicited suddenly in response to tactile stimulation to the gums or teeth, the resulting increased tone in the jaw and cheeks frequently occurs concurrently with attempts to release the stimulating agent. It commonly occurs together with strong flexor patterns of the neck, shoulder girdle and arms.

Tongue thrust

A tongue thrust is a very forceful protrusion of the tongue from the oral cavity, so strong that it interferes with normal feeding patterns, whatever the age of the client.

Chapter 2: Respiration and Aspiration

INTRODUCTION

Martin *et al* (1994) state that breathing and swallowing functions of the respiratory and digestive systems 'appear reciprocal and well co-ordinated in the healthy adult'. This chapter aims to emphasise the value of considering respiratory problems within case history taking and functional assessment, as well as promoting the importance of multidisciplinary team (MDT) working, in order to prevent the occurrence of aspiration pneumonia.

NORMAL RESPIRATION

This section (based on Warland, 1997) will cover (a) basic lung anatomy, (b) lung histology and physiology, and (c) the cough reflex.

Basic lung anatomy

The diaphragm is the main muscle of inspiration (see Figure 2.1). Situated below the lungs, it moves down and out, increasing the thoracic volume and decreasing intrathoracic pressure. Thus air is drawn in through the mouth or nose, pharynx and trachea.

The lungs are made up of progressively smaller airways that terminate in air sacs or alveoli (see Figure 2.2), where oxygen can diffuse into the blood stream. If the

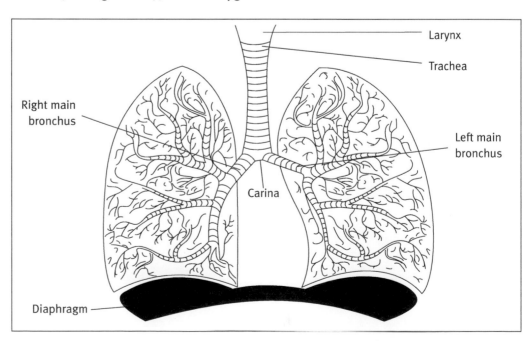

Figure 2.1
The lower respiratory tract

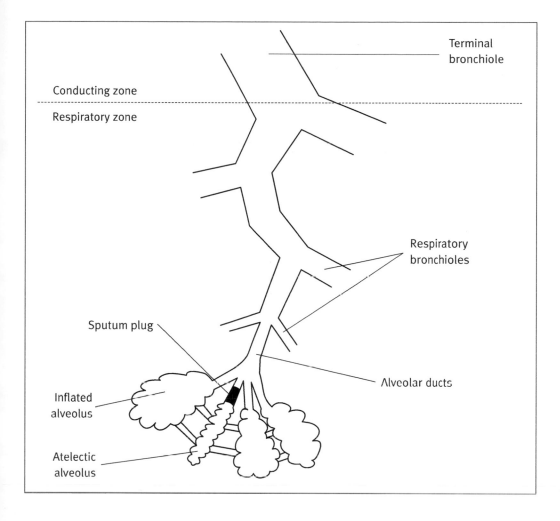

Figure 2.2
Details of the lower respiratory tract

airways are blocked the alveoli will collapse and be unable to participate in gas exchange. Small channels exist between the alveoli, allowing air to pass from alveoli to alveoli directly. This allows re-inflation of a collapsed (atelectic) alveolus, which will facilitate removal of the blockage. This is the basis of many physiotherapy treatments. If sputum retention occurs and a sufficiently large breath is inhaled, these channels re-inflate the collapsed alveoli and will promote removal.

The angle of the right main bronchus as it leaves the trachea is less acute than the left. 'The right bronchus, therefore, is the more common pathway for aspirated material' (Dikeman & Kazandjian, 1995), entering the apical segment of the lower lobe.

Lung histology and physiology

The trachea and lungs are lined with pseudostratified ciliated columnar epithelium interspersed with mucus-secreting goblet cells and submucus glands (see Figure

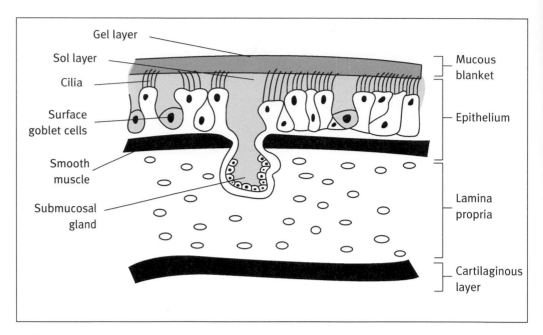

Figure 2.3
Histology of the lung

2.3). Small particles that escape filtration in the nose are trapped on the sticky mucociliary carpet and are then moved, by cilia, against gravity, from the bronchioles to the throat over a period of several hours. This carpet moves secretions to the pharynx and larynx, from where the debris is swallowed or, if excessive, expectorated. Between 10ml and 100ml of secretions are produced every day, potentially rising to 300ml or more in the presence of infection or disease. This process is known as the mucociliary transport mechanism.

The cough reflex

Sputum clearance depends primarily on mucociliary transport and secondarily on the cough. A cough can clear secretions from the sixth or seventh branch of the tracheobronchial tree.

The normal reflexive cough has four phases. First, irritation stimulates receptors located in areas within the oropharynx, larynx and lung tissue. This stimulus provokes impulses in the cough centre in the brain. Deep inspiration leads to compression of the air, consisting of reflex glottic closure and forceful contraction of the expiratory muscles, which results in a rapid rise in pleural and alveolar pressures. Expulsion occurs when the glottis suddenly opens and the air, as it explodes outwards, shears secretions from the airway walls. The nasopharynx is closed off, resulting in the foreign bodies being expelled via the mouth.

Coughing is accompanied by violent swings in intrapleural pressure and blood pressure, which potentially may cause long segments of distal airway collapse. These normally reopen with a deep breath, but if the individual is unable to take a deep breath they may stay closed for lengthy periods.

RESPIRATORY PROBLEMS

Respiratory function is affected by:

- Smoking. It is important to note that many individuals report an increase in mucus production (and hence the need to expectorate) approximately two weeks after giving up smoking. This is caused by the mucociliary transport system returning to normal after the long-term effects of smoking.
- Dehydration
- High inspired oxygen concentrations
- Hypoxia
- General anaesthetics
- Atmospheric pollutants
- Interruption by endotracheal suction
- Infection – the cilia become overwhelmed by mucus
- Existing lung disease, for example chronic obstructive pulmonary disease (COPD), tumour, asthma
- Immobility
- Ageing
- Very high alcohol levels
- Poor positioning, which will affect lung volumes

COPD is a group term for chronic bronchitis, emphysema and asthma. One of the major causes of COPD is smoking; hence clients may present with coexisting cardiovascular disease. Causes of asthma include genetic and environmental factors and, unlike COPD, it is normally treatable.

Neurological disorders, such as stroke (CVA) may alter the cough reflex (see below), irrespective of the presence or absence of dysphagia.

THE EFFECT OF SWALLOWING ON NORMAL RESPIRATION

Selley *et al* (1990) reported that the complex respiratory patterns associated with feeding in normal adults mature 'in the teenage years'. While this feeding–respiratory pattern (see Figure 2.4) may be altered voluntarily, it will be repeated in 95 per cent of swallowing events assessed in a non-dysphagic individual. The swallow–breath pattern can be described as follows:

◆ Exhalation ceases before spoon/lip contact and inspiration occurs during contact;

◆ In 93 per cent of swallows, expiration is followed by apnoea;

◆ Apnoea occurs during the middle and late oral phase of swallow, and hence precedes laryngeal elevation;

◆ Total apnoeic interval averages approximately one second. There is not a significant increase in the duration of the apnoeic pause with small increases in bolus volume (3ml, 10ml and 20ml), but there is a significant difference in the duration of the apnoeic pause with a large volume (a 100ml straw swallow);

◆ An expiratory burst normally follows the period of apnoea;

◆ There is a positive correlation between duration of laryngeal elevation and duration of the apnoeic pause;

◆ Respiration returns to normal between mouthfuls;

◆ A large volume, 100ml straw swallow is likely to result in several uninterrupted swallows, and a higher occurrence of post-swallow inspiration.

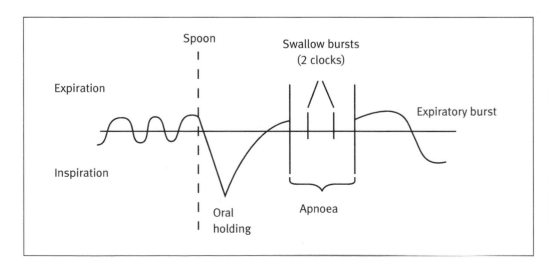

Figure 2.4
The swallow–breathing pattern

THE EFFECT OF RESPIRATORY PROBLEMS ON SWALLOWING

COPD and asthma cause more shallow, irregular respiration, to the extent that anticipation of a utensil touching the lips may be enough to set off a cough. Clients with COPD may demonstrate decompensations in airway protection at the level of the larynx and reductions in swallow efficiency. This is related to characteristic mouth breathing; slow prolonged bolus preparation; laboured lingual motility; prolonged ascent and closure of the larynx (possibly due to the low rest position of the larynx and reduced elasticity of the tracheolaryngeal complex); alterations in apnoea onset or offset; premature reopening of the larynx and resumption of respiration; and diminished respiratory defence mechanisms (Martin *et al*, 1994). In addition, those with COPD frequently require more calories, which may be difficult to achieve in view of the above alterations to the normal swallow pattern, with or without a coexisting dysphagia.

ASPIRATION

Definitions

Definitions of penetration and aspiration were introduced in Chapter 1. To recap, penetration is material penetrating the laryngeal vestibule; aspiration is material entering the airway below the vocal folds. Both penetration and aspiration may occur before, during or after the swallow, and a swallow need not be triggered for either to occur. Aspirated material includes food, drink, saliva, medication, foreign bodies and refluxed gastric contents.

Normally aspiration that occurs before the swallow is due to a disorder in tongue movement or a delay in triggering the swallow. Reduced glottic closure potentially results in aspiration during the swallow. If residue remains in the pharynx after the swallow, it may enter the airway during respiration. Causes include poor base of tongue movement, pharyngeal wall weakness and reduced laryngeal movement.

Aspiration in the healthy conscious subject is not usual, although it is not uncommon for normal adults to aspirate saliva during sleep. Some 70 per cent of clients with depressed consciousness have been found to aspirate.

Silent aspiration occurs when the respiratory mechanism does not respond in any audible way to the aspiration event. That is, there is no cough or throat clear. Logemann (1998) has estimated that 40 per cent of clients silently aspirating are missed on bedside evaluation.

Aspiration pneumonia: causes and consequences

Causes of aspiration pneumonia

Aspiration does not necessarily result in aspiration pneumonia. Terpenning (1994) suggests that the defences against aspiration pneumonia are oral, pharyngeal and pulmonary. Even if the invader breaches these defences it still must find a way to establish a camp in the lung and begin to proliferate before the client will develop an aspiration pneumonia. This tough pulmonary host defence mechanism is a complex series of events that is not completely understood or predictable.

Langmore *et al*'s (1998) recent study produced the most comprehensive investigation of the causes behind the development of aspiration pneumonia in the elderly. Overall she found that dysphagia was not of high predictive value in the development of aspiration pneumonia. The most significant predictive factor was dependency on others for feeding, particularly in nursing home residents (typically bed-bound) with decayed dentition or who rarely brushed their teeth. Poor oral hygiene is of significance if oral secretions containing anaerobic bacteria are aspirated, or if they are aspirated alongside food or drink. While bacterial flora in the oropharynx can be altered by severe underlying disease, inactivity or malnutrition, a more direct cause of altered colonisation in the oropharynx is the presence of oral or dental disease. Plaque, gingivitis, periodontal disease and tooth decay will alter the flora within the mouth, and could change the bacterial composition of saliva. Reduced salivary flow increases the concentration of bacteria in the saliva. The presence of tube feeding is also a risk factor, possibly because of the aspiration of oral secretions or reflux of the gastric contents.

Nash (1988) described how tracheostomies increase the incidence of aspiration, by fixing the trachea to the anterior neck skin. This in turn causes reduced elevation and anterior movement of the larynx, allowing food and/or secretions to enter the partially unprotected airway. The cough is less effective because of the tracheostomy, and the client becomes desensitised owing to chronic air diversion through the tube.

In an earlier study, Langmore *et al* (1994) highlighted the importance of medical diagnosis as an indicator in the development of aspiration pneumonia. In her elderly population, COPD was the highest indicator (29 per cent), then a neurological diagnosis (25 per cent), followed by CVA (13 per cent). Likelihood increases further with multiple medical pathologies.

Dysphagia was found to be of greatest effect in an acute hospital caseload. Solid food can cause obstruction of large airways, which may then lead to disruption of gas exchange due to atelectasis (collapsed alveoli). Small amounts of clear liquids should not in themselves cause a problem unless the pH is very high or low, or they are ingested in sufficient volume to cause asphyxia.

Reflux is a potential side effect of nasogastric or gastrostomy tube feeding (see Chapter 9 for detail of these feeding methods). In addition, the presence of a nasogastric tube may diminish the sensitivity of the gag reflex so that the potential for aspiration is further increased. Langmore did not find an association between reflux (see below) and the development of pneumonia, unlike Terry and Fuller (1989). Aspiration of large amounts of acidic gastric contents may result in an acid burn to the lungs, causing adult respiratory distress syndrome (ARDS). Gastric contents are normally acidic, but may become alkaline if medication is employed (see 'Reflux' below). Bacteria can only live in more alkaline gastric contents, resulting in potentially infectious complications if aspiration occurs.

Consequences of aspiration pneumonia

The effects of aspiration on health are difficult to predict (Rosenbek *et al*, 1996). The clinical symptoms that develop are dependent on (a) the frequency of aspiration, (b) the quantity and nature of the aspirated material, and (c) the underlying host response.

If pharyngeal contents enter the airway, and are not cleared spontaneously by coughing, a wide range of pulmonary symptoms may result. Terry and Fuller (1989) report that pulmonary consequences of aspiration can be severe. Most frequently pneumonia occurs. Airway obstruction may be caused by particulate material. Repetitive aspiration may cause diffuse scarring in the lung, leading to bronchiectasis, the main symptom of which is increased sputum production. The most troublesome and consistently fatal consequence of aspiration is ARDS, which is characterised by the onset of severe respiratory distress, hypoxia and chest x-ray studies that show diffuse bilateral infiltrates, indicating damage throughout the lungs.

Diagnosis of aspiration pneumonia

Signs and symptoms in the elderly can be subtle and atypical, differing from those seen in younger patients. De Paso (1991) suggested that, if using the term 'aspiration pneumonia' (sometimes called Mendelson's syndrome), the clinician needs to define precisely the type of material aspirated, using the term 'pulmonary aspiration of . . . '.

While research studies use strict criteria to diagnose pneumonia (for example, elevated white blood cell count, fever, and new infiltrate on chest x-ray), in clinical practice the following are used as signs and confirmation of aspiration:

◆ Observation of cough and voice quality

◆ Spiking temperature (a sign of infection)

◆ Suspicion with certain medical diagnoses, such as neurological disorders

◆ Raised respiratory rate

◆ Dyspnoea (a rapid and shallow breathing pattern, involving the accessory muscles)

◆ Pallor

◆ Sputum sample analysis (sent for culturing, this may be found to contain traces of food and/or drink, as well as pathogens)

◆ Increased amount of sputum

◆ Darker coloured sputum

◆ Right base of lung signs on auscultation (stethoscope) and/or chest x-ray

◆ Reduced blood oxygen saturation and altered arterial blood gases

Management of aspiration and aspiration pneumonia

This section draws on Warland (1997). Prevention is better than cure. Comprehensive assessment by the speech and language therapist (in conjunction with the MDT) aims to identify the risk of aspiration, directing the clinician to appropriate preventative management. This is the subject matter of this manual. Management should also include training members of the MDT regarding feeding and swallowing problems (see Chapter 13), pressing for appropriate nutrition and hydration to maximise host resistance (see Chapter 9), and promoting the importance of dental services for clients (see Chapter 6).

If aspiration pneumonia occurs, it is essential that the client be sufficiently hydrated to prevent secretions becoming too thick to expectorate. Airway humidification using inhaled moisture is also employed.

Medical management of aspiration pneumonia includes antibiotic treatment to reduce infection, and analgesia to prevent pain interfering with client expectoration of secretions. Medical intervention such as bronchoscopy (for areas of lung collapse which prove unresponsive to physiotherapy) or thoracotomy (to remove solid obstructions, for example a peanut) may be necessary in extreme conditions. In conjunction with drug treatment of aspiration pneumonia, a range of physiotherapy treatments are utilised, including postural drainage (gravity facilitated movement of mucus from the distal to the proximal region); manual techniques (percussion and vibration); breathing techniques to promote collateral ventilation (that is, promoting the opening of the small channels which exist between the alveoli), and encouraging and assisting coughing.

REFLUX

Authors are divided on whether reflux is of significant predictive value for the development of aspiration pneumonia (see above). Aspirating gastric contents may masquerade as the consequences of a swallowing disorder. Often, however, the two go hand in hand: the client is unable to swallow safely, and therefore is given tube feeding which results in reflux combined with difficulty coping with saliva, potentially coupled with oral hygiene problems.

While the cricopharyngeal sphincter can normally prevent refluxed material entering the pyriform fossae, large volumes may cause an increase in pressure, which may overwhelm this sphincter, potentially leading to aspiration. The oesophagoglottal closure reflex (aryepiglottic approximation and vocal fold adduction) provides a level of protection to reflux, in response to abrupt oesophageal distension. This reflex relies on an intact brainstem response.

Reflux management

A number of techniques are available for reflux management, depending on diagnosis of the underlying cause:

◆ Posture: sitting up or lying on the right side to promote gastric emptying;

◆ Medication: for example, antacids form a 'raft' that floats on the surface of the stomach contents to reduce reflux and protect the oesophageal mucosa; ranitidine reduces acid production; metaclopramide stimulates gastric emptying; cisapride increases gut motility;

◆ Tube feeding: for example, reducing the speed at which the feed passes through the tube; only feeding the client during the day, when sitting at an angle of 40 degrees or more.

INTRODUCTION

This chapter is concerned with the subjective assessment of feeding and swallowing. It is divided into nine sections:

1　Aims of assessment

2　Pre-packaged assessments

3　Case history

4　Bedside or clinical observations

5　The relationship between body posture, tone and oromotor control

6　Cognitive factors

7　Oral and oral preparatory stage assessment

8　Pharyngeal bedside assessment

9　Hierarchy of consistencies and quantities

AIMS OF ASSESSMENT

The purpose of performing a functional assessment of swallowing is to establish the presence or absence of a swallowing disorder, and to avoid potential complications of dysphagia. First, if dysphagia is present, the clinician will want to establish whether it is safe for the client to proceed with oral intake and, if so, what will be recommended. Second, the clinician will want to establish whether the client is able to meet their nutrition and hydration needs orally. We suggest that clinicians ask themselves the following questions:

a　Is the client

◆　At risk of aspiration on fluids? If so, on what consistencies (for example, thick, thin), and how severe is the risk?

◆　At risk of aspiration on foods? If so, on what consistencies (for example, soft diet, mixed textures and stringy or crumbly foods), and how severe is the risk?

◆　At risk of not meeting their hydration needs orally, and how severe is the risk?

◆　At risk of not meeting their nutrition needs orally, and how severe is the risk?

b What stage(s) are involved, oral and/or pharyngeal and/or oesophageal, and is the overall impairment mild, moderate or severe?

c What may be the hypotheses for the cause, recovery pattern and duration of the dysphagia? Can a tentative prediction of prognosis for the short and long term be made?

d Will the client benefit from referral to other professionals for further evaluation: for example, to a dietitian or ENT surgeon?

e Will the client benefit from intervention and, if so, what type?

This information can then be shared with the client, family and multidisciplinary team, and an appropriate management plan developed.

It may be that the results of the assessment identify the client's swallowing mechanism as intact. 'Not because they are old' (Health Advisory Service 2000, 1998), an independent enquiry into the care of older people on acute wards in general hospitals, identified various reasons for older people experiencing weight loss and dehydration. These included staff not recognising that the person may require help with positioning in a chair; not being able to reach food placed on a tray or table on the opposite side of their bed; needing assistance to feed themselves physically owing, for example, to visuospatial difficulties; food being taken away too soon; prescribed feeding aids not being provided at meals. Naturally, the management suggested by the speech and language therapist to the care staff will be directed towards staff education and training regarding positioning food and drink appropriately, and offering assistance with these where necessary.

PRE-PACKAGED ASSESSMENTS

Before describing in detail the content of both subjective and objective assessments, it is useful to consider a small number of pre-packaged assessments. Published assessments include those for screening (that is for identifying at-risk clients or those who have dysphagia), and evaluations aiming to provide a differential diagnosis (that is, defining the anatomic and/or physiological disorder so as then to provide a therapy and management plan). The latter is the aim of this manual.

'A Screening Procedure for Oropharyngeal Dysphagia' (Logemann, et al 1999)

This is a 28-item screening test used for identifying those clients who aspirate, have an oral stage disorder, a pharyngeal delay or a pharyngeal stage disorder. Screening items are presented in five categories: medical history variables, behavioural variables, gross motor variables, observations from oro-motor testing, and observations during swallow trials. The results direct the clinician to diagnostic testing, eg bedside assessment, cervical auscultation, and videoendoscopy. The low specificity means that a patient at high risk of aspiration is guaranteed a diagnostic study, while patients without aspiration will potentially receive an unnecessary diagnostic evaluation.

'Dysphagia Evaluation Protocol' (Avery-Smith et al, 1997)

This protocol and accompanying pocket manual, devised by occupational therapists, aims to provide a 30-minute swallowing assessment. It considers factors that may contribute to a swallowing problem, and provides guidelines for conducting a bedside swallowing evaluation. The results of this evaluation may help to determine whether or not a client requires videofluoroscopy or alternative assessment procedures.

'A Functional Assessment of Dysphagia' (FAD) (Kennedy, 1991)

The FAD aims to provide a comprehensive evaluation package for circumstances where a modified barium swallow (videofluoroscopy) is either inaccessible or inappropriate. It was developed for use with adults who are neurologically impaired, with acquired swallowing disorders. The assessment begins with a preliminary checklist to give an overview of the patient's condition. It moves on to an orofacial examination before proceeding to direct evaluation of the swallow pattern on a variety of consistencies. The client's responses are recorded on a five-point rating scale, which is item specific with weighting for each being equal (Kennedy *et al*, 1993). The FAD forms the basis of the assessment material detailed in this text, with modifications following further developments in research and clinical practice.

'Paramatta Hospital's Assessment of Dysphagia' (Warms et al, 1988) and 'Chicago Clinical Evaluation of Dysphagia' (Cherney et al, 1986)

Although these two protocols continue to be used in the UK, we suggest that the recent bedside assessments of Avery-Smith and Logemann will become increasingly popular in years to come. 'Paramatta' and the 'Chicago' provide useful summaries of the dysphagia assessment, particularly of the oral and oral preparatory stages.

CASE HISTORY

This section will focus on the importance of the history obtained from (a) the medical referral and medical notes, where available, and (b) the client and carers' report.

As with any clinical work, investing time in seeking out background medical information and taking a thorough case history from the client can be invaluable. This enables the clinician to formulate and modify a hypothesis prior to, during and after the bedside assessment or clinical evaluation. Asking appropriate questions at this stage will enable the clinician to select only those relevant aspects of the bedside assessment, reducing client fatigue. Only then can the most appropriate management be decided upon: whether there is the need for a more detailed objective assessment, or direct or indirect management strategies.

The type and style of case history will depend on the type of client and the setting in which they are seen. This in turn will determine the management and training needs of the client, their family, staff and any other carers. Naturally, the needs of a client and their 'team' in an acute unit are different from those of an outpatient with a progressive degenerative disease, or an adult with a learning disability in a residential home.

Background medical information

Aetiology

Some of the known causes of dysphagia are given below. These have been divided into neurological causes, mechanical causes, medication-induced dysphagia, psychogenic dysphagia and odynophagia (painful swallowing). Prior medical complications, and those which may arise as consequences of dysphagia, exacerbate swallowing problems.

Responsibility for diagnosis of neurological causes usually rests with the neurologist; mechanical causes are the province of the otolaryngologist or, in the case of dysphagia affecting the oesophageal stage, of the gastroenterologist. Reports from the relevant speciality are the essential basis for informed and selective assessment of dysphagia. Whenever diagnosis of the underlying cause is uncertain, insights from any member of the investigating team may contribute to successful interpretation. Where possible, the current and past medical history are obtained from the referral request and medical notes. These may provide information regarding the onset and duration of the swallowing problem; the presence, type, duration and method of placement of any device to facilitate breathing, such as intubation, tracheostomy or ventilator; and the presence, type and complications of any oral or non-oral nutrition.

If, from the history, it is clear that the patient has an infection, muscle wasting, injury or systemic illness that increases their metabolic requirements, it is especially important that they receive prompt and adequate nutrition and hydration to facilitate recovery. This demonstrates how medical history affects on management.

Neurological causes

A list of some of the neurological causes of dysphagia is given below. An explanation of the less common causes is provided in brackets.

◆ Alzheimer's disease and other dementias
◆ Achalasia (failure or incomplete relaxing of the lower oesophageal sphincter, resulting in retention of food in the oesophagus)
◆ Acute botulism (toxin can affect neuromuscular junction of cranial nerves to laryngopharynx)
◆ Bulbar poliomyelitis (infection involving neurones of the brainstem)
◆ Cerebral palsy

- Cerebrovascular accident, CVA or stroke (see below for details)
- Diabetes (long-standing, insulin-dependent diabetes can increase the severity or prolong the recovery period of dysphagia because of the potential for myopathies and neuropathies)
- Encephalitis
- Guillain-Barré disease
- Huntington's disease
- Meningitis
- Motor neurone disease
- Multiple sclerosis
- Myasthenia gravis (autoimmune disorder of the neuromuscular junction involving pharynx and/or larynx, swallowing worsens during a meal and late in the day)
- Myotonic dystrophy (progressive disease characterised by hypertonicity of muscles with a delay in release of muscle contraction, reflux may be experienced)
- Neurosurgery
- Oesophageal reflux
- Oesophageal spasm
- Oesophageal sphincter dysfunction
- Parkinson's disease
- Polymyositis (results in muscle inflammation, weakness and pain)
- Polyneuropathy (or peripheral neuropathy as seen in diabetes)
- Scleroderma (a neuromuscular disease involving connective tissue with atrophy and fibrosis of smooth muscle, which may affect the oesophagus)
- Trauma
- Tumours
- Wilson's disease (a disorder of copper metabolism that results in diffuse damage to the brain and liver; both pharyngeal and oesophageal stages may be impaired)

It is significant to note (a) the location of the lesion affecting the brain following a stroke, and (b) any history of previous strokes resulting in bilateral or multiple lesions, as these affect management and prognosis. Logemann (1998) provides the following descriptions of swallowing disorders, which result from the different lesion sites.

In the initial weeks following a brainstem stroke, the pharyngeal swallow may be absent, and the oral stage may be functional. Characteristics after the swallow returns are delayed pharyngeal swallow, unilateral pharyngeal paresis, reduced laryngeal elevation, reduced cricopharyngeal opening, and unilateral adductor vocal fold paresis. In many cases, the more severe the stroke, the longer the recovery period.

In the case of cortical strokes (that is, those affecting the cerebral cortex), the swallow is usually functional in three weeks. With a left hemisphere stroke, the predominant impairment is of the oral stage. There may be swallow apraxia, delay in initiating the oral swallow, mild delay in pharyngeal triggering, and a usually normal pharyngeal swallow. Right hemisphere strokes tend to compromise the pharyngeal stage, resulting in aspiration. There may be mild oral transit delay, mild delay in triggering the pharyngeal swallow, and mild slowness in elevating the larynx. Often these clients have difficulty integrating therapy or compensatory strategies into oral feeding, including the chin-down position (see Chapter 6), because of cognitive impairments and relative inattention. This explains why clients with right hemisphere strokes may take longer to resume and increase their oral intake than those with left hemisphere strokes.

In subcortical strokes the swallow is usually functional within three to six weeks of the onset. Characteristics of this type of stroke are mild oral transit delay; greater delay in triggering the pharyngeal swallow than in a cortical stroke, and general weakness in the pharyngeal swallow. The manifestations of the latter are reduced laryngeal elevation, reduced tongue base retraction, and unilateral pharyngeal weakness.

Finally, clients who have had bilateral or multiple strokes often have a higher incidence and greater severity of swallowing abnormalities (Horner *et al*, 1988; Horner *et al*, 1993). Oral stage difficulties may include repetitive tongue movements and prolonged oral transit times of five seconds or more. Pharyngeal problems include reduced laryngeal elevation and glottic closure resulting in penetration, and unilateral pharyngeal weakness leading to pooling in the pyriform sinus on the affected side. As with clients with right hemisphere strokes, their attention may be reduced, and so they have difficulty utilising strategies and focusing on the task of eating and swallowing. The increased severity of dysphagia may be a result of the mechanism not having returned to normal after the first stroke.

Structural or mechanical causes

- Burns (from inhalation of hot smoke or ingestion of caustic agents)
- Candida albicans (fungal infection in oropharynx and/or oesophagus)
- Cervical osteophytes (bony outgrowths of the cervical spine)
- Cervical spine displacement
- Chronic obstructive pulmonary disease (see Chapter 2)
- Fibrosis (scarring following surgery or radiotherapy)
- Lupus (inflammatory connective tissue disorder affecting skin and internal organs, and causing inflammatory changes in muscle)
- Obstruction (for example, abscess, tumour, physical object)
- Oedema or acute inflammation to oral mucosa or aerodigestive tract
- Oesophageal impaction
- Oesophageal stricture
- Oesophageal web
- Pharyngeal pouch
- Surgery (for example, to the cervical spinal cord, damage to the recurrent laryngeal nerve post thyroid or cardiac surgery)
- Sjorgren's syndrome (an autoimmune disease associated with salivary hypofunction resulting in oral stage dysphagia)
- Tracheostomy tube (see Chapter 8)

Blitzer (1990) states that caustic agents may produce oesophageal dysmotility (see the section below on medication-induced dysphagia), and aspiration due to decreased sensation and fibrosis. The latter two changes may be irreversible and difficult to treat, requiring gastric surgery.

Assessment and management of surgical causes, including laryngectomy, glossectomy, reconstruction of the jaw and changes to these areas as a result of radiotherapy, are not within the remit of this book.

Medication-induced dysphagia

Stoschus and Allescher (1993) explain how dysphagia can be caused by the following:

a The normal side effect of a drug which can affect
- Smooth or striated muscle function of the oropharynx or oesophagus (for example, tricyclic antidepressant, antipsychotic or neuroleptic drugs)
- The dryness of the oral mucosa (caused, for example, by anticholinergics such as atropine, hyoscine; antiemetics; antihypertensives; antiarrythmics; diuretics and opiates)

b A complication of the therapeutic action of a drug, such as oral and oesophageal fungal infections developing in clients requiring immunosupressive drugs

c Medication-induced oesophageal injury, as a result of prolonged contact of a potentially caustic drug (for example, alendronate) with the oesophageal mucosa. This is most common in the elderly and is promoted by taking the medication (particularly at night) without enough fluid.

In addition, they note that acute and chronic alcohol use can cause oesophageal dysmotility. Finally, oxygen given via a facemask can also cause xerostomia (dry mouth, which can be painful).

Psychogenic dysphagia

Emotional distress and disturbance, such as grief, loss of social contact at meals, anxiety, depression and, sometimes, denial often accompany dysphagia. However, there is a sub-group of patients with dysphagia who complain of swallowing difficulties, such as reduced appetite, reduced food intake, altered food selection patterns (restricting themselves to soft, easily liquefied food), altered oral sensation and activities associated with the oral preparation. There may be a history of recurrent episodes of difficulty swallowing. Clients may report the sensation of a lump in the throat, or pain at the level of the larynx (globus pharyngeus), which is present continually and not merely during swallowing. It can give rise to fear of an imagined obstruction, which they locate at the level of the cricopharyngeal sphincter.

On examination, there is no evidence of neurological abnormality. There can be visibly increased levels of musculoskeletal tension and, on palpation, the larynx may be perpetually held in an elevated position, resulting in pain. Videofluoroscopy may be performed to exclude the possibility of obstruction. The results may reveal abnormalities in the oral stage and an essentially normal pharyngeal stage.

Research by Barofsky and Fontaine (1998) suggests that these clients have higher levels of anxiety, interpersonal sensitivity and depression when compared to other clients complaining of dysphagia. Once this diagnosis has been made, the clinician provides strategies to facilitate lower levels of musculoskeletal tension in the jaw, tongue, pharynx and larynx.

Odynophagia

Hendrix (1993) defines this as painful swallowing, especially if the pain is described as 'sharp', usually indicating ulcerative lesions of the pharynx or oesophagus. If the pain is described as 'dull' or 'squeezing', it is usually associated with oesophageal spasm.

The client and carer's report

Identify the site of the problem

Logemann (1998) states, 'studies have shown patients who are aware a disorder is present to be highly reliable in their identification and description of a swallowing disorder'. Edwards, in the 1970s, showed that clients with dysphagia were able to identify the site at which the problem was localised with a high degree of accuracy.

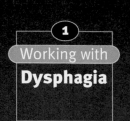

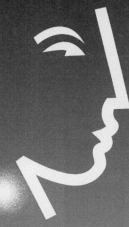

SWALLOWING ASSESSMENT QUESTIONNAIRE

Name of client
_____

Date of birth
_____

Date of assessment
_____

Seen alone/with
_____

Name (and designation) of informant
_____

HISTORY OF THE PROBLEM

Do you have a problem with eating and drinking?
_____

Does it cause you concern or distress?
_____

When did the problem start?
_____

Can you briefly describe the problem?

_____

Did it start gradually or suddenly?
_____

Is it getting better, worse or staying the same?
_____

What would you say was the cause?

_____

Have you found any 'tricks' that help?
_____

MEDICAL INFORMATION

Are you taking any medication at the moment? If so, what?

_____

Have you had any chest infections in the last year?
_____

If so, how many?
_____

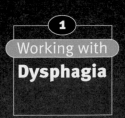

SWALLOWING ASSESSMENT QUESTIONNAIRE

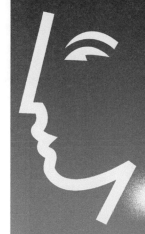

Have you had any urinary tract infections in the last year? If so, how many?

_____

Have you had any previous lung or breathing problems (for example, asthma, emphysema, chronic obstructive pulmonary disease)?

_____

Do you smoke cigarettes?
_____

Do you think your voice has changed (for example, become hoarse, quieter, whispery) in the last year?

_____

Have you had any previous swallowing or ENT problem?

_____

Do you have any pain on swallowing (for example, referred pain in the ear)?

_____

WEIGHT, NUTRITION, HYDRATION AND PILLS

Have you lost weight?
_____

How much?
_____

Since when?
_____

Does your food need special preparation before you can eat it (for example, cutting up into small pieces, mincing, liquidising)?
_____

Do you avoid certain foods because they are difficult to swallow or you dislike them?

_____

Can you list them?

Photocopiable

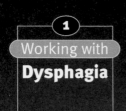

SWALLOWING ASSESSMENT QUESTIONNAIRE

Have you found any tricks that help your swallowing?

Do you have difficulty swallowing pills?

Do you ever need help to eat or drink?

Do you prefer to eat in company or alone?

How long does it take you to eat a meal?

Do you finish your meals?

Do you feel hungry after eating?

How many cups of tea and glasses of water or juice do you drink in a day?

Do you enjoy eating and drinking?

What did you have to eat and drink yesterday, and was that typical for you?

ORAL STAGE

Does saliva dribble from your mouth?

Do you have difficulty keeping food or drink in your mouth?

Is it hard to take food off a spoon or drink from a cup?

Is chewing difficult?

Do you find food left in your mouth after swallowing?

Does it get left in your cheeks or stuck to the roof of your mouth?

Do you need a drink to wash down mouthfuls?

Do you need to swallow more than once?

Do liquids ever come back through your nose when you swallow them?

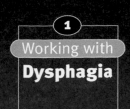

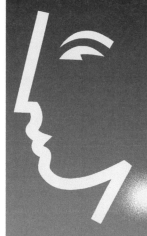

SWALLOWING ASSESSMENT QUESTIONNAIRE

PHARYNGEAL STAGE

Do you regularly wake up at night coughing? (This can indicate reduced triggering of the swallow reflex, resulting in saliva pooling in laryngopharynx or acid reflux that stimulates a cough reflex)

Do you cough or splutter when eating or drinking? If so, how often?

Does food or drink ever go the wrong way, into your windpipe? If so, how often?

Do you need to take care when you eat or drink in case things go the wrong way?

Do you ever feel that food gets stuck? If so, where?

OESOPHAGEAL STAGE

Do you ever feel that food gets stuck further down, in your gullet?

Do you get pain behind your breastbone after swallowing?

Does food, drink or acid ever come back up your throat?

NOTES AND ADDITIONAL INFORMATION

A useful starting point on meeting the client is to ask them, 'Why are you here today?' and 'What would you like me to do?' This can establish their perception of the problem and their expectations of the clinician. Following this, more specific questioning can take place using a questionnaire such as the one above. The clinician should be sensitive to the client's economic, cultural, educational and employment background when asking questions.

BEDSIDE OR CLINICAL OBSERVATIONS

Before performing the clinical dysphagia examination, it is necessary to observe the client and the environment. In hospital, it is often invaluable to observe the client from the nurses' station. We suggest that the following areas be assessed.

Level of alertness

Can the client maintain an alert state, or do they become drowsy? How do they react to the clinician's entrance? Are they drowsy but rousable to verbal stimuli? Are they unrousable to verbal or gentle tactile stimuli? This information can help the clinician decide whether the client is able to participate in the clinical dysphagia examination at that time, or whether it would be beneficial to return later when they are more able. If they are drowsy, or their levels of alertness fluctuate constantly during the day, it is possible that their nutrition and hydration needs will be compromised.

Communication and cognition

Is there evidence of dysphasia, dysarthria, dyspraxia, cognitive change or dementia? Do they have difficulty participating owing to one of the above rather than reduced alertness? Can they follow commands, do they need non-verbal cues, are they able to maintain their attention, and do they fatigue easily? These have implications for management.

Caregiver–client interaction

Are the client and the carer aware of the swallowing problem, or do they deny its presence? Is the client motivated to participate in the clinical dysphagia examination? The clinician should respect the client's wishes if the client is not willing to participate.

Auditory and visual acuity

If the client usually wears a hearing aid or requires glasses, the clinician should ensure that these are available and in good working order.

Posture and movement

The ideal position for a client (see Figure 3.1) to participate in a clinical dysphagia examination is sitting in a chair, maintaining an upright and symmetrical posture with the head slightly flexed (see later section, 'The Relationship between Body Posture, Tone and Oromotor Control'). It is important to establish the best possible position for the client before commencing the assessment and it may be helpful to ask for assistance from other members of the multidisciplinary team, such as physiotherapists, occupational therapists or nurses. During the evaluation the clinician may wish to trial the use of different head postures to reduce the risk of aspiration (see Chapter 7). This may be compromised by neurological impairment and fatigue. Clients who are unsafe to sit in a chair will need to sit as upright as possible in bed. If the client with dysphagia is a 'walkie-talkie' (a term coined by Groher and Crary, 1997 to describe clients who are able to walk into an outpatients clinic, for example), they are less likely to experience pulmonary complications.

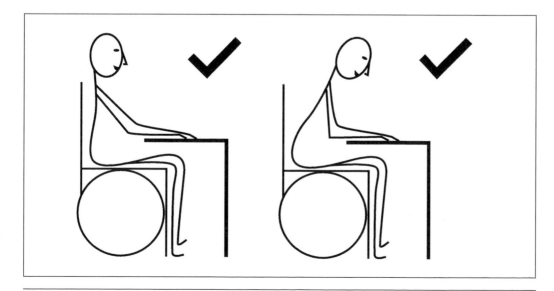

Figure 3.1
Ideal posture involves symmetry: an extended or upright trunk, upright head with chin tuck, flexion at the hips and knees, with both feet flat on the floor

Respiratory status

The client may have aspiration pneumonia and pulmonary complications at the time of assessment (see Chapter 2). We suggest that the clinician takes time to observe the client's breathing pattern at rest, and to note any abnormal noises or patterns such as noisy or rattling upper airway sounds, whether the rate is normal, rapid, or fluctuating, or if there are periods of apnoea (suspension of breathing). If there is any respiratory distress, it may not be appropriate to proceed with the assessment. This allows the clinician to compare the client's baseline respiratory rate with any changes during the clinical dysphagia examination. Chronic obstructive pulmonary disease (COPD) may be one cause of mouth breathing, which may indicate shortness of breath due to difficulty maintaining the oxygen saturation of the blood. The presence of oxygen given via a facemask or nasal prongs suggests pulmonary or cardiac involvement.

Coughing

It is helpful to ask other members of the multidisciplinary team if they have observed the client coughing spontaneously. Clients who cough often during the day, or who report regularly waking at night because of coughing, may be experiencing less frequent triggering of the swallow reflex. This results in saliva pooling in the laryngopharynx, triggering a cough reflex. Repositioning a client in bed or in their chair may also elicit a spontaneous cough reflex. The clinician should note the strength of this.

Structural abnormalities

Groher & Crary (1997) suggest that the clinician observe movement of the client's valves: that is, the lips, jaw, tongue, velum and larynx. These can be assessed during conversation. The clinician should note any facial asymmetry; whether the client is able to maintain lip seal; if there is evidence of velopharyngeal incompetence resulting in hypernasality and the presence of dysphonia. Signs of previous surgical intervention to head and neck; the presence of prostheses and dentures and their retention will be commented on. Langley (1988) states that 'Clients with neurological disorders often have difficulty tolerating their dentures, or, if tolerated, in holding them in place. Retention depends on normal tone in the muscles of the cheek; if tone is weaker on one side, the dentures will shift towards that side. Denture fixative and alterations to the denture itself are only effective in preventing this if the underlying problem is subject to improvement.'

Diet and hydration

The clinician should note the presence of, and client's reaction to, intravenous drips, feeding tubes, catheters, and food or drink on the table or locker. If the client is eating or drinking or being fed, we suggest that general comments be made about the oral and pharyngeal stages. A basic comment on the client's nutrition status may be made if there is severe wasting and minimal subcutaneous fat. If the client is dehydrated, their oral mucosa and skin may be dry. Urinary tract infections (UTIs) are more common when an individual is dehydrated. If they have a catheter bag and it is visible, the colour and consistency of the urine may indicate dehydration (dark yellow and syrupy) or infection (cloudy, darker yellow-brown). Clients with a UTI may have foul-smelling urine. Dehydration can lead to thick and tacky saliva.

Oral hygiene

Foul mouth odour can be caused by a variety of digestive tract conditions, not just those affecting the mouth. The clinician should observe how clients manage their own secretions. Do they swallow spontaneously or drool? Food or fluid residue in the mouth or on their clothes indicates difficulties self-feeding, and with the oral stage. Poor oral hygiene can contribute to the development of fungal infections such as candida, where the tongue may become bright pink or seen in the form of white – creamy-coloured plaques on the surface of the tongue. In clients whose immune systems are compromised, for example people with AIDS, or those receiving radiation and/or chemotherapy, 'the lesions of herpes or Candidiasis may be so extensive and slow to heal as to seriously interfere with nutrition' (Hendrix, 1993). Candida can spread down to the larynx and oesophagus, resulting in dysphonia, compromised airway protection and oesophagitis. Aspirating infected saliva, which may be tenacious and contain anaerobic bacteria, fungal spores and flora, can lead to pulmonary complications (see Chapters 2 and 6).

THE RELATIONSHIP BETWEEN BODY POSTURE, TONE AND OROMOTOR CONTROL

The purpose of this section is to give an appreciation of the importance of appropriate positioning of clients to facilitate swallowing in the clinical dysphagia examination, and in management of the swallowing problem. First, consider how every part of the body is connected. It is not appropriate therefore, to view the mouth in isolation.

Postural stability

In order to develop and sustain normal patterns of movement, we require a stable base from which to develop movement. Without postural stability, mobility may become less controlled or sometimes impossible. This stability allows us to achieve movement of our limbs, head, neck, fingers, toes, jaw and tongue. Stability is achieved by the balance of contraction in agonist and antagonist muscles around joints. Postural stability is sustained by normal muscle tone. As we move through space, we rely on proprioception – the internal feedback that allows muscles to know what they are doing. The vestibular system provides information about changes in posture and gravity and therefore balance. In summary, to make fine or gross motor movements we rely on postural stability, normal muscle tone, proprioception and balance.

An activity to experience postural instability

Sit in a chair with both feet lifted off the floor. Tip to one side so that you are sitting on one buttock. Experience the sensation of trunk imbalance. Notice the compensations made throughout the muscles of the body. Now imagine being fed in this position. Would it be easy to maintain coordinated movements for swallowing? What is it that allows you to compensate so well?

Abnormal tone

After insults to the central nervous system (CNS) or the peripheral nervous system (PNS), there may be changes in muscle tone, depending on the aetiology. Increased

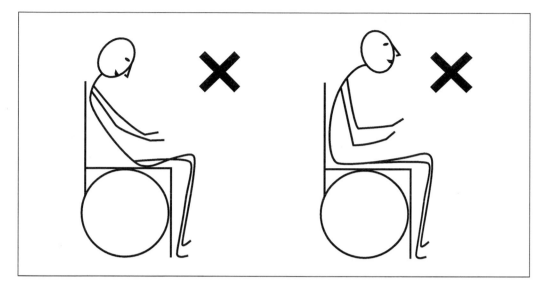

Figure 3.2
Head flexion: unstable posture with curvature of the trunk and without the stable base of the hips and feet

muscle tone results in spasticity. Decreased muscle tone results in flaccidity. As abnormal tone increases, postural defects occur. An increase in spasticity can result in flexion. Postural defects can affect head position, which in turn affects the action of bringing the hand to the mouth and swallowing. Abnormal head position may affect lip closure, jaw closure, control of bolus, the ability to inhibit tongue thrust, laryngeal movement, palatal movement and transfer of the bolus to the pharynx.

The head extended up and back is associated with an open jaw position, poor lip closure, tongue thrust and difficulty initiating the trigger of swallow reflex. Conversely, a flexed head position is associated with improved lip seal, reduced tongue thrust, prompter swallow trigger and increased palatal movement (see Figure 3.2).

We suggest that where possible, clinicians aim to achieve the following for their clients, in assessment and management of swallowing problems:

◆ Symmetry
◆ Optimal tone
◆ Postural stability
◆ Inhibition of spasm
◆ Slightly flexed head
◆ Extended trunk
◆ Flexed hips and knees
◆ Independence

COGNITIVE FACTORS

This important area is often neglected and, while information must be gathered during both case history taking and observation (see above), it is also worthy of special consideration. Clients with dysfunction at the pre-oral ingestion stage are normally unaware of their problems and have difficulty providing a history.

Cognitive skills may be impaired owing to a number of acute and/or chronic factors. Identifying the aetiology of the cognitive impairment will influence whether the assessment proceeds at that time, or whether it would be more appropriately deferred until an acute cause has been remediated. For example, poor nutrition, hydration and acute infections, such as a urinary tract infection, may significantly affect cognition. The resulting dysphagia may be resolved with appropriate treatment of the underlying cause. Conversely, the client with a known diagnosis of dementia must be assessed with this in mind. It is vital to remember that an acute and chronic cause may coexist.

Factors to consider include the following:

◆ *Strategies*: has the client spontaneously applied any, and if so are they beneficial? Have they retained those given by previous therapists? What form of prompt is required – verbal, visual, and/or written?

◆ *Supervision*: what level is required to ensure that strategies are implemented? For example, one-to-one, or passive 'keeping an eye on' in the dining room.

◆ *Fatigue and stamina:* frequently fatigue and poor stamina are the result of neurological impairment or poor nutrition.

◆ *Level of alertness and attention*: how long can this be maintained – for a few mouthfuls, or a full meal? Is the client easily distracted?

◆ *Awareness of food or drink*: this includes recognition of food, drink and utensils (however, for some cultural groups it is normal to eat with the fingers).

◆ *Self-feeding*: is the client able to self-feed or do they require hand-on-hand feeding? Are they totally dependent?

◆ *Fear and confidence regarding eating and drinking*: is this at an appropriate level in relation to the assessment findings?

Can these problems be remediated, or is their impact too great for eating and drinking to be safe and sufficiently effective to meet the individual's nutritional and hydration needs?

ORAL AND ORAL PREPARATORY STAGE ASSESSMENT

Assessing sensation

This section considers (a) essential points relating to observation of swallowing reflexes, particularly hypersensitivity and the emergence of primitive and/or abnormal reflexes, (b) oral sensation, and (c) taste.

Swallowing reflexes

Throughout the assessment of the oral stages, and earlier in the case history, the clinician will be alert to identify any reflex behaviour that may interfere with effective swallowing. Such reflex behaviour is categorised as normal sensation, hypersensitivity of the normal reflexes, pathological or abnormal reflexes, and the re-emergence of primitive reflexes.

In the neurologically impaired, reflex activity may be stimulated by:

◆ Food, drink, saliva and other orally ingested material

◆ Emotional stimuli, such as stress

◆ Inappropriate posture

The pathological and primitive reflexes are most commonly seen in clients with bilateral hemispheric or frontal lobe damage.

Normal reflexes: the cough, swallow and gag

Further detail relating to the cough and swallow can be found in Chapter 1 'The Normal Swallow', and below in the pharyngeal assessment section. Only these two reflexes will be intentionally elicited during an assessment.

A gag reflex is normally triggered by a noxious or foreign stimulus in the posterior oral cavity or pharynx. These stimuli would include material refluxed from the oesophagus, vomit, a finger, or other solid items which have not been subject to oral preparation. Food does not normally trigger a gag. The gag is characterised by a sudden and strong contraction of the pharyngeal walls, soft palate and larynx to squeeze and eliminate the foreign substance. It is now generally agreed that the gag reflex is not a useful indicator of aspiration (Bleach, 1993), therefore we suggest that it is not appropriate to test this in a functional assessment. It is unpleasant for the individual, and potentially for the clinician. In addition, the variation in sensitivity between normal healthy adults is vast, and can be influenced by anticipation and level of alertness. If the gag is elicited in error during an assessment, the therapist will aim to determine (a) whether this was appropriate to the context, and (b) if sensation is normal or whether the client is hypersensitive.

Hypersensitivity

This generally relates to the gag reflex, but one must be aware of the large range of sensitivity between and within normal individuals. As a result it may be difficult to define normal sensitivity, but a rule of thumb would be that hypersensitivity is indicated if the gag is triggered during the oral preparatory phase (assuming no gastrointestinal problems), so that it interferes with the normal swallowing process.

Pathological or abnormal reflexes

When working inside the mouth beware of stimulating a bite reflex or a tongue thrust. A bite reflex is defined as involuntary biting with difficulty releasing. It is abnormal at any age and elicited by touching lips, teeth, gums or tongue blade. Ask the nursing team about their experiences during routine mouth care and, whatever their report, remember always to proceed with caution. If a tongue thrust is present, the bolus may be pushed out of the mouth by the tongue, and it may be difficult to achieve sufficient oral nutrition. Many readers will have observed this reflex in clients with cerebral palsy.

The primitive reflexes

The primitive reflexes are normally present in infancy, but disappear with maturation and as cortical control develops. In adults they are normally inhibited by the higher centres of the brain, suggesting the level of impairment should they reemerge. They may interfere less with swallowing than the pathological reflexes, and in some cases can be used to assist in the management of dysphagia. Further detail is provided in Chapter 1.

Oral sensation

Remember to ask the client about this first if possible, as they may be able to provide you with the information and so make it unnecessary to carry out the assessment detailed below. If required, it is possible to assess oral sensation and muscle tone simultaneously, using a gloved finger dipped in water (see Chapter 11, 'Health and Safety' regarding appropriate gloves). Remember to compare the affected side with the unaffected side, particularly for tone.

It is important to proceed with care: have members of the multidisciplinary team noted a bite reflex or hypersensitive gag during mouth care, suctioning or oral feeding?

Areas to assess are the following:

◆ Buccal muscle and orbicularis oris tone. Tightness indicates increased tone, flaccidity reduced tone. It is essential to compare the affected and unaffected sides to get an impression of normal tone, before confirming the presence of increased tone.

◆ Food residue in the lateral sulci which indicates reduced sensation and tone. This has implications for oral hygiene and the potential aspiration of pooled material.

◆ Ridges on the inside of the cheek, where unintentional biting has occurred as a result of reduced sensation.

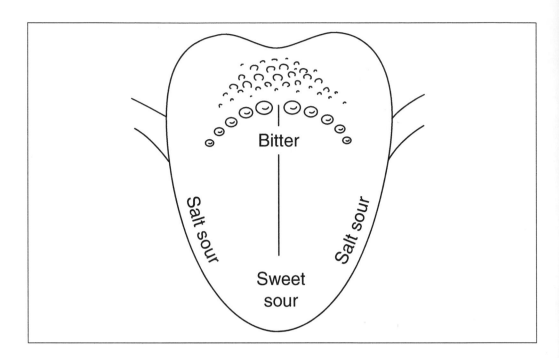

Figure 3.3
Distribution of taste sensors on the tongue

Taste

Again, ask the patient about whether their perception of taste, and hence potentially their enjoyment of food, has been affected. Patients occasionally report a burning sensation in their mouth. We suggest that the clinician checks for any localised infection (information regarding oral hygiene is to be found within 'Oral Stage Management', Chapter 6).

Taste can be evaluated by asking the patient to identify salt (salt solution), sour (lemon juice), bitter (quinine) and sweet (sugar solution) flavours, which can be applied to the appropriate area of the tongue (Figure 3.3) with a moistened cotton swab.

Assessing taste may not be the priority during the functional swallowing assessment, but it may be utilised (a) to help elicit a dry swallow, particularly a sour bolus, and (b) to provide information regarding intact sensory innervation; bitter is distinguished via cranial nerve IX; the other tastes are identified via cranial nerve VII. Management may also be aided by taste, as the following:

◆ General stimulation, such as for those in a low state of consciousness

◆ Providing pleasure for clients who are 'nil-by-mouth'

◆ Desensitisation for clients with head injuries

◆ Clients with multi-system degeneration who often enjoy highly spiced food

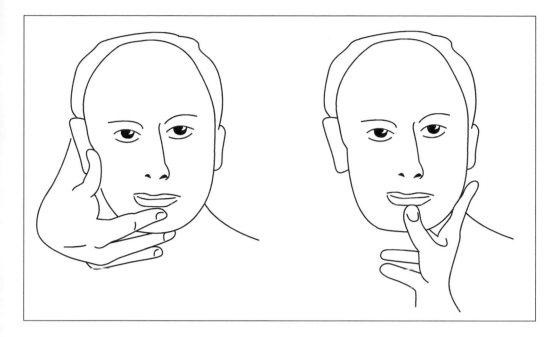

Figure 3.4
Two techniques for facilitated jaw closure

Assessing specific oral movements

Ideally, the oral movements are viewed during eating and drinking, but if necessary they can be assessed in isolation. Assessing specific oral movements in isolation is functional when simulating movements involved in eating and/or drinking. Modelling may be necessary for those with receptive language impairments, and it is essential to check that the foods/fluids utilised do not conflict with the client's dietary or religious requirements, eg gelatine in fruit pastilles and marshmallows. Always observe for a dry swallow (by asking the client to swallow their saliva) if possible.

Jaw movement in chewing

Create a chew bag, offering food (such as a fruit pastille, piece of banana, or a piece of marshmallow) wrapped in double thickness moist cotton gauze (10cm x 10cm). Place the food in the centre of the gauze, bring the corners together and twist to keep the food firmly in place. Keeping hold of the end of the bag, place it between the client's teeth on one side and ask them to chew. Jaw closure can be facilitated with support if necessary (see Figure 3.4).

Tongue protrusion

Ask the client to lick jam placed on the lips or from a spatula held in front of the mouth. If using a wooden spatula, first wet it with water as the dry wood can stick to the delicate mucosa of the tongue and cause discomfort.

Lateral tongue movement

The most effective means of assessing the figure-of-eight movement in isolation is to provide something for the tongue to move from side to side. Varying diameters of suction catheter are available to make the task easier or more difficult. (We suggest that you ask a hospital physiotherapist for a variety to trial yourself.) Alternatives include strawberry or liquorice shoelaces, or the chew bag described above. Asking the client to lick jam or chocolate from each corner of their mouth, from inside their cheeks, or around their gums (although not the figure-of-eight) can also help you to assess lateral tongue movement.

Tongue tip elevation

Apply a sticky substance such as chocolate (spread or a moistened chocolate button) to the anterior palate and alveolar ridge. Ask the client to lick it away.

Anterior to posterior tongue movement

Roll up a 10cm × 10cm cotton gauze square into a sausage shape. Dip this into a coloured liquid such as blackcurrant juice, diluted methylene blue (see Chapter 8) or food colouring. Squeeze out a small amount of the liquid so that it does not drip, then lay the gauze along the tongue, positioning it as far back as possible. Keeping hold of the end, ask the client to swallow. Normal tongue movement is indicated if the removed gauze shows (a) a central groove, (b) a 'hump' resulting from contact between the tongue and hard palate, and (c) a lighter area at the sides where the tongue and molars produced a seal.

Lip seal

Lip seal, and strength of seal, can be assessed in isolation. Ask the client to grip and hold a dampened spatula between the lips, or to hold a Polo mint (moistened) tied with dental floss, between the lips. Resistance can be applied in both situations.

PHARYNGEAL STAGE BEDSIDE ASSESSMENT

To aid clarity, the detail of each aspect of pharyngeal stage assessment is provided separately. In reality, whatever aspect of the swallow is being assessed, the clinician will be gathering evidence of pharyngeal skills and/or problems in parallel.

A study by Logemann (1993) indicated that 40 per cent of subjects who regularly aspirated on videofluoroscopy were identified as safe by bedside assessment alone. Objective pharyngeal assessments will be discussed later, but while they are increasingly available for all patients, including those managed in the community, a significant quantity of information can be gathered from the bedside assessment, as will be discussed. The reader is referred to Chapter 2 ('Respiration and Aspiration') before commencing this section.

Cough reflex

As previously discussed, this vital reflex is required for airway protection and to expel material from the larynx and upper airway. The sensitivity and the effectiveness of the cough reflex are the key aspects to note.

The easiest client to assess is one taking oral intake, who was noted by the referring agent to be coughing on food and/or drink. The assessment can then determine the following:

◆ What consistencies of food and/or drink cause the problem.
◆ When the cough is triggered: before the swallow, immediately after, after some delay, only after a build-up of residue in the larynx (as evidenced by a gurgly voice – see below), only on food, only on drink, or never, despite evidence of pooled material.

◆ The effectiveness of the cough. Is the penetrated/aspirated material cleared quickly by a strong or weak cough, or by one that is more similar to a throat clear, which takes some time to remove the material? Is the cough ineffective, resulting in an inability to clear the material at all?

To gather more specific information regarding a client's cough, the clinician may utilise the following techniques, which it may be appropriate to integrate into a client's management. The clinician may test the *voluntary cough* by asking the client to cough. Alternatively this can be modelled for the client. However, it is important to demonstrate the cough while turning the head away from the client to minimise the possibility of droplet infection. A *reflexive cough* is produced in response to an irritant, mirroring the normal response to aspirated/penetrating material. The clinician's thumb can act as an irritant using a 'tracheal tickle'. This may be tested by pressing toward the trachea at the sternal notch, with a circular movement, until a cough is stimulated.

For clients with tracheostomies, information on the cough is normally available from the nursing staff or physiotherapists, who can advise on how far the suction catheter enters the airway before a cough is elicited.

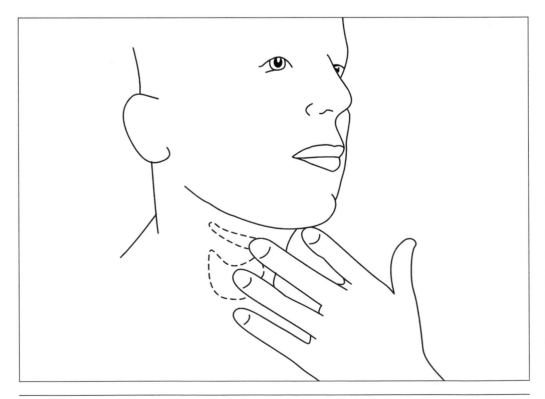

Figure 3.5
Tactile assessment of the swallow

The swallow reflex

In an assessment, the client is often asked to swallow to command: that is, to swallow their saliva. For many clients, including those with cognitive and/or language impairment, this is a difficult response, even if the clinician models the target behaviour. Recent research into the single 'command' swallow (see Chapter 1) indicates that it is different from the sequential swallow we employ for food or drink. A dry swallow to command does, however, provide information about the swallow in a controlled environment and could be used therapeutically (see Chapter 7).

For many years, tactile assessment of swallowing (see Figure 3.5) was considered a standard pharyngeal stage assessment technique. Recently, however, it has been suggested that manual assessment using this three-finger test interferes with swallowing physiology.

We suggest that the swallow reflex be assessed initially by observing and listening. The three-finger test can then be introduced if the client is sufficiently prepared for tactile assessment and able to tolerate it without interference to their normal swallow pattern. The three-finger test can be a useful tool to teach carers, and may enhance client awareness of the swallow (for example, delay, number of clearing swallows).

Whichever techniques are employed (and this includes objective pharyngeal stage assessments), observe for the following:

◆ A quick laryngeal elevation, with slightly slower descent.
◆ The extent of elevation.
◆ Tongue pumping (felt with the index finger on tactile evaluation), which often occurs together with laryngeal bobbing (repetitive elevation and descent, but elevation is incomplete).
◆ Effort to initiate a swallow reflex.
◆ Possible delay in triggering the swallow: up to three seconds is generally considered sufficiently safe, whereas over five seconds may indicate a higher risk of aspiration. Time alone should not be an indication of safety, however. A significant delay with particular consistencies (see below) and no evidence

of aspiration/penetration may be acceptable if it means that a client can continue with oral intake (see Chapter 6, 'General Issues in Management', for further discussion).

◆ Clearing or 'check' swallows. Remember that individuals without swallowing difficulties may require one or more clearing swallows, particularly on stickier or crumbly consistencies. Of concern are multiple clearing swallows that do not appear to clear residue (oral and/or pharyngeal), and which potentially cause rapid fatigue.

This evaluation of the swallow reflex requires that the oral and oral preparatory stages be relatively intact. It is possible to assess the pharyngeal swallow in isolation, although its functional significance is questionable. A 10ml syringe is filled with 1ml chilled water and 9ml air. The clinician fires the syringe quickly at the client's posterior pharyngeal wall. The chilled water hitting the posterior pharyngeal wall causes prompt contraction of the pharynx against the base of the tongue and the triggering of a swallow reflex. Considerable skill and practice is required to ensure accuracy. It is well worth practising this on colleagues first.

Voice quality

Two aspects of voice quality are important to assess. The first is wetness, often described as a 'gurgly voice'. A wet voice quality indicates pooling of the bolus in the pyriform fossae (unilateral or bilateral) which has spilt over into the airway, penetrating the vocal folds. This pooled material may subsequently be aspirated if the larynx is insensitive to it.

The aim is to identify the cause of this pooling. For example, clients with later stage Parkinson's disease (and those with cognitive impairment) typically present with a wet voice in conversation owing to a build up of saliva in the oral cavity that has not triggered a swallow reflex. The saliva overspills the base of the tongue and the valleculae. It may then pool in the pyriforms and above the larynx. Because of reduced laryngeal sensation they are not aware of it, producing a wet voice quality. Yet with food and/or drink, there may be no evidence of aspiration. For the majority of clients with dysphagia, however, a wet voice quality pre- or post-swallow indicates a risk of aspiration.

Of greatest importance are a client's ability (a) to clear the pooling spontaneously, and (b) to employ and learn strategies to clear residue from the larynx.

Monitoring voice quality can be a useful management strategy (see later chapters). Wet voice quality can be assessed by talking to the client during the clinical evaluation, or by using the following strategy:

1 Client puts chin down.
2 Food or drink is given.
3 Place fingers on client's larynx to feel for the swallow.
4 Ask client to say, 'ahhh'. Listen for wet voice quality.
5 If it is present, ask client to cough to clear it. Repeat from stage (4). NB: if the client is unable to clear wet voice quality by coughing on three occasions, the food/drink trials should be abandoned.
6 If it is not present, repeat from stage (2).

The second aspect is breathy quality or hoarseness, which may indicate impairment of vocal fold adduction, although the degree of vocal fold and false vocal fold closure in swallowing may still be sufficient to avoid penetration or aspiration. Unilateral and bilateral vocal fold weaknesses often occur together with pharyngeal weaknesses, the latter potentially resulting in pooling (see below) and hence a wet voice quality as discussed above. Where dysphonia persists and shows little or no sign of resolving itself, referral to an ear, nose and throat (ENT) surgeon for evaluation of vocal fold function is indicated, in order to rule out vocal fold pathology. This is particularly important where the client has progressed in other areas of rehabilitation, but their dysphonia remains unchanged.

Patient reports of pooling

As already cited, Logemann (1998) states that 'studies have shown patients who are aware a disorder is present to be highly reliable in their identification and description of a swallowing disorder'. The client who may be able to indicate the site of pooling by pointing to the area or side of the neck (valleculae indicates poor base of tongue movement; pyriform fossae indicate pharyngeal weakness; posterior wall of pharynx indicates a pharyngeal constrictor problem) will normally have devised strategies to clear the problem, with varying degrees of effectiveness. Clients who have no, or limited, awareness of pooling were discussed earlier. Further information on pooling is available from objective assessments (see below).

HIERARCHY OF CONSISTENCIES AND QUANTITIES

Clinicians working with clients who have dysphagia are aware that controlling the consistency and quantity of a bolus is essential in their management. Information regarding the normal swallow, factors affecting the swallow, and assessment of the oral, oral preparatory and pharyngeal stages, is amalgamated in this section.

We suggest that the following basic principles be considered before the assessment commences:

◆ *Unit policies and professional body guidelines.* At the end of this section, we will provide a range of options for a hierarchy, which may not be in line with readers' local policies. Erring from such policies may have professional and legal consequences (see also Chapter 10). This hierarchy is provided as a guide only.

◆ *Health and safety.* Issues of key significance are legislation regarding food storage, preparation and handling (see Chapter 11).

◆ *Level of experience and expertise.* If in doubt, seek supervision and/or a second opinion.

◆ *Current fashions and trends.* Sections of this text may become out of date, so the authors stress the importance of maintaining an up-to-date knowledge of current research in assessment and management.

◆ *Client fatigue.* It may be necessary to skip steps without compromising client safety to ensure that the evaluation does not fatigue the client unnecessarily (see the section on cognitive factors above).

◆ Hiiemae and Palmer (1999) report that the assessment of swallowing using a 'command swallow' model does not demonstrate normal physiology, except for liquids.

The theory underpinning modification of consistencies and quantities is provided below.

Thickening fluids

Water loses its cohesion after one second. Therefore, if a client's swallow is delayed, the risk of penetration and/or aspiration increases significantly. Thickened fluids move more slowly, providing the individual with more time to initiate a swallow. A number of thickening agents are commercially available, normally by prescription (see Pulver, 1999, for evaluation of thickening agents currently available in the United Kingdom). Alternatively, drinks that are naturally thicker may be utilised, such as tomato juice, pulpy fruit juices (for example, mango), yogurt drinks, thick milk shakes and some liquid supplements available on prescription (for example, Ensure).

Liquid viscosity can range from normal, to very thick, through to set, using thickeners. A scale might be normal → syrup → thick syrup (still pourable) → thick milk shake (McDonalds restaurant style) → set.

Chilling (foods or fluids)

A cold or chilled bolus is effective in stimulating a delayed swallow. See Chapter 12, 'Health and Safety', for advice regarding ice.

Purée versus soft, easy chew foods, versus normal food consistencies

Purée may appear to be a safer consistency as the initial feeding programme for a client with dysphagia, but there are problems in its use, and normally it can be superseded by soft, easy chew foods, or even normal consistencies moistened with gravy, custard, cream and so on. Arguments against the use of purée include (a) it has a tendency to be nutritionally incomplete; (b) it is not a normal texture for most people, (c) it is difficult for individuals to differentiate the various tastes they are given, and (d) there is a tendency for carers to mix portions of purée together. Purée is of value, however, for the cognitively impaired client who experiences difficulty suppressing chewing in order to swallow, or for those who spit out lumps. If these problems do not exist, the cognitively impaired client will fare best with a familiar, normal consistency. Examples of soft, easy-to-swallow foods are provided in Appendix I. This topic is discussed further in Chapter 9.

Bolus size

Information is provided in Chapter 1 Factors affecting the normal swallow, and in the discussion regarding pooling, above.

Carbonated drinks

It has been suggested (Nixon, 1997) that carbonation facilitates faster oral and pharyngeal transit times; decreases the incidence of pooling and penetration, and improves laryngeal elevation, decreasing the incidence of aspiration when compared with non-carbonated thin fluids. Fizzy drinks may heighten a person's awareness of the bolus in the oral cavity, increasing the speed of initiation of the swallow reflex. Carbonated drinks are normally drunk chilled, which may add to their stimulating effect (see above). Clients may be more accepting of fizzy drinks (because of their normality) than of thickeners. Since they are normally sweet, there are increased potential problems if aspirated, and there are implications for oral health (see Chapter 6). Carbonated fluids may be most suitable for those experiencing milder problems, such as penetration.

Self-feeding

The significance of self-feeding is outlined in Chapters 1 and 2. Information regarding utensils and crockery can be found in Chapter 9.

A guide to a hierarchy of consistencies and quantities is provided (Scenario 2). If problems are identified at any stage (see Figure 3.6), the clinician should form a hypothesis regarding the cause of the problem, and then implement and evaluate strategies (see above).

Scenario 1

'Where a client is already taking some food/liquid orally, speech and language therapists should observe him/her drinking and/or eating, provided it is not contraindicated by clinical examination' (RCSLT, 1996). A client's normal mealtime would therefore appear to be the most appropriate situation in which to assess this group. There may, however, be a limit to the number of mealtime observations a clinician can fit into their working day, and the availability of suitable foods at other times may be restricted.

Scenario 2

A small step progression is presented. We suggest that a minimum of two presentations of each consistency be assessed. It is worth considering that the initial mouthfuls may be a problem owing to the impact of disuse–dysfunction (see Chapter 1).

1   Perform oral hygiene using (sterile) water on a pink foam stick or toothbrush (see Chapter 6).

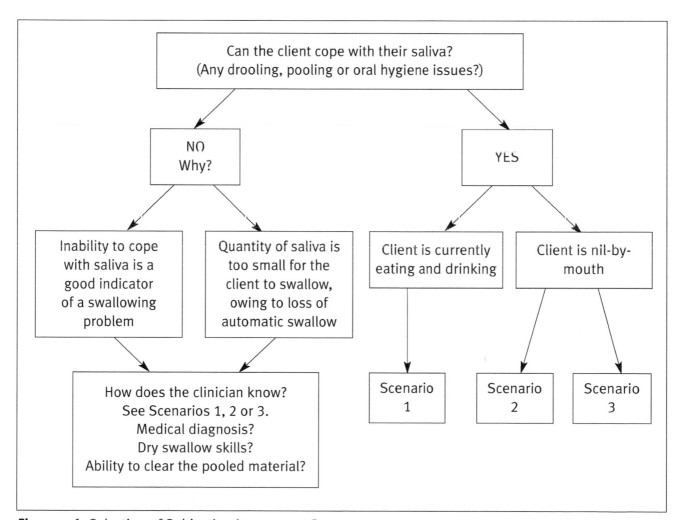

Figure 3.6 *Selection of Subjective Assessment Routes*

2 One teaspoon of crushed ice/'slush' (ideally made from sterile water). Use cold fluids/foods to increase stimulation.

3 Half a teaspoon of water.

4 Whole teaspoon of water.

5 Sips of water (with hand-on-hand assistance).

6 Sips of water (without assistance).

7 Semi-solids and/or thickened liquid (see above, re consistencies).

8 Chewing (bread for example).

Scenario 3

This scenario is more contentious, but is required frequently in the real world, where the consistencies required for the initial stages of the hierarchy above are often unavailable. Cognitively impaired clients may also benefit from the presentation of normal foods and/or fluids. Foods which may be readily available and suitable include:

◆ Ice-cream

◆ Yogurts/mousses

◆ Chilled supplements – fluids or pudding consistencies (see Chapter 9)

◆ Cereals, such as Weetabix

Ice-cream, yogurt or mousses are frequently available on wards or from the catering department, or an appropriate consistency can be bought en route to a client's home. They are chilled and soft. Any management programme based on the assessment will then be possible for the staff or carers to replicate when reintroducing oral intake, ensuring that information regarding spoon sizes (for example, teaspoon) and portion size are provided. Counter-arguments regarding the use of ice-cream include the speed at which it melts in the mouth to become a thin fluid/mixed consistency which, if aspirated, may be more likely to lead to aspiration pneumonia than water.

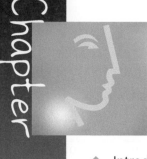

Chapter 4: Objective Assessment

INTRODUCTION

'A limitation of clinical examination is that the information on the pharyngeal stage of swallow can only be inferred and "silent" aspiration may go undetected. Findings from clinical assessment should be confirmed using a complementary technique when there is any doubt about management' (Scottish Intercollegiate Guidelines Network, 1997).

The focus of this chapter is the indications and procedures for use of the following instrumental techniques to study swallowing: videofluoroscopy, fibre-optic endoscopic evaluation of swallowing safety (FEESS), cervical auscultation, pulse oximetry, scintigraphy, electromyography and surface electromyography (SEMG), ultrasound imaging and manometry. Before any of these assessments are performed, the therapist will carry out a clinical dysphagia examination, in order to be familiar with the client. The use of these techniques requires specialist training. 'Practitioners must maintain and enhance their knowledge and skills on a regular basis, by attendance at appropriate meetings, Special Interest Groups and conferences' (Guidelines for speech and language therapists for endoscopic evaluation of the vocal tract and radiological imaging, RCSLT, 1999). The results obtained contribute to the making of a diagnosis, and guide the subsequent management approach.

VIDEOFLUOROSCOPY

Purpose

Currently this radiological examination (also known as a modified barium swallow) is the most commonly used and reliable adjunct to the bedside or clinical dysphagia assessment. It evaluates the swallow anatomy and physiology; identifies the patterns of bolus flow; shows impaired physiology (for example, reduced laryngeal elevation and cricopharyngeal opening), and the consequences of this impaired physiology (for example, aspiration, residue). Logemann (1998) states that it should not be conducted for the sole purpose of determining whether or not a person aspirates. Instead, it is used when the results of the clinical dysphagia examination are inconclusive, in order to 'enable commencement of some manner of safe, efficient oral intake immediately, in the context of achieving daily nutritional and hydration requirements and a safe swallow'. It aims to confirm the symptoms described by the client and identified by the clinical dysphagia assessment, and allows the evaluation of the usefulness of treatment strategies. For this reason Groher and Crary (1997) prefer to call it the 'rehab swallow'. They state that its purpose is 'to determine the need for and the direction of swallowing rehabilitation'. It is invaluable in educating clients and carers, as it can demonstrate the nature and severity of the problem. This is especially true for individuals with a likely diagnosis of a psychogenic dysphagia, or those who deny that aspiration occurs.

Candidates

All clients receiving this investigation need to have undergone a thorough clinical dysphagia assessment first. This is in order to identify clients for whom this investigation is not appropriate and thus avoid unnecessary exposure to radiation. The procedure may be undertaken on clients who are alert and possess sufficient cognitive awareness to complete the study. It may be used with people with a stable, progressive or recovering medical condition, to confirm a diagnosis of psychogenic dysphagia or to investigate unexplained symptoms from the clinical assessment. However, in our opinion, it is only suitable for the more robust individual. We suggest that clinicians ask themselves, 'Will it benefit the client's management and functional outcome?'

Procedure

The assessment involves using a fluoroscopy machine, video recorder, microphone and, ideally, a counter timer. Generally the speech and language therapist performs this procedure with a radiologist and radiographer, who are knowledgeable regarding radiation safety and techniques (see Chapter 11). The radiologist has primary responsibility for making a medical diagnosis and for identifying masses and structural deviations, particularly in the oesophageal stage and gastric region, which a speech and language therapist is not qualified to do. 'The speech and language therapist will normally take responsibility for ... evaluating and interpreting function in conjunction with the radiologist' (Guidelines for

Radiological Imaging, RCSLT, 1999). It can be helpful to have a physiotherapist or nurse present who can assist with achieving optimal positioning and suctioning where necessary. Specialised seating equipment may be required.

The speech and language therapist provides pertinent information to the radiologist regarding the client's medical history, and relevant information about their cognitive, nutritional, hydration and respiratory status. Results of previously completed assessments will be shared (Radiological Imaging, RCSLT, 1999). It is usual to commence in the lateral plane, examining the anatomy for any abnormalities (for example, the cervical vertebrae for osteophytes, valleculae, tongue base and airway entrance), and watching for any movement disorders, such as tremors.

There are two approaches to the protocol: either it can be individualised, or it can be stereotyped (fixed order of presentation of specific volumes and viscosities). The former is unique to the client's swallowing skills and uses familiar foods and utensils. Their usual carer presents the food, commencing with the safest consistency. In contrast, Logemann's protocol (1993) suggests giving measured amounts of liquids in the same order – that is, 1ml, 3ml, 5ml, 10ml and then drinking from a cup. Paste or soft purée is presented next and then, finally, a solid bolus such as biscuit. Three trials of each consistency are provided.

We suggest that both thin and thick fluids be assessed using 1ml and 5ml from a spoon, followed by 10ml from a cup and then free cup drinking. Where possible, the clients feed themselves to make the swallow physiology as normal as possible. We try always to use the same consistency of mousse, yogurt or fromage frais, mixed with the same quantity of barium powder, to prevent variation between people who prepare the food. This can then be spread on to a biscuit. If it is felt this consistency is too crumbly for the client, a sponge muffin can be dipped into liquid barium and then presented to the client.

If it is likely that the client will aspirate on barium liquid or a semi-solid containing barium powder, it is preferable to use an alternative such as the radio-opaque liquid, Omnipaque. This is because barium, though inert, may set solid in the lungs and cause pulmonary complications. Omnipaque, if aspirated, is an irritant to the lungs, causing copious coughing. However, it is usually absorbed by the lungs without serious pulmonary consequences. Finally, the radio-opaque liquid, Gastrograffin, commonly used to detect fistulae in the digestive tract, is not recommended for use where there is any risk of aspiration as it can lead to respiratory arrest if aspirated.

What to look for in the lateral view (Logemann, 1998)

As the swallow is initiated, watch the bolus movement.

◆ Does the bolus hesitate?
◆ If so, where and for how long?
◆ Where is the bolus head when the pharyngeal swallow is triggered?
◆ Does any bolus enter the airway before, during or after the pharyngeal swallow?

Observe

◆ Oral tongue movement, bolus consolidation and transfer
◆ Palatal closure
◆ Onset of laryngeal elevation as a sign of triggering the pharyngeal swallow
◆ Airway closure
◆ Cricopharyngeal opening (this occurs almost simultaneously with airway closure)
◆ Tongue base movement towards the pharyngeal wall and anterior movement of the posterior pharyngeal wall.

Immediately after the swallow, identify the location of residue and define its cause.

◆ If it is in the oral cavity, go back and review the pattern of oral tongue movement.
◆ If it is in the valleculae, go back and review the pattern of tongue base and pharyngeal wall movement.
◆ If it is in the pyriform fossa, go back and review the laryngeal elevation and cricopharyngeal opening.

◆ If it is on the pharyngeal walls, go back and review the pharyngeal wall contraction.

Observe for any aspiration of residue below the vocal folds, and the client's reaction to aspiration, penetration or residue. Rosenbek *et al* (1996) suggest an eight-point penetration–aspiration scale, which has intra- and inter-judge reliability. This can facilitate more precise reporting as it allows the clinician to note how far into the airway the material passes, and whether or not it is expelled.

What to look for in an anterior–posterior view

Indications to obtain an anterior–posterior view are

◆ Abnormal physiology leading to asymmetry and/or weakness and hence residue or aspiration
◆ Client history suggesting pharyngeal asymmetry – that is, neurological deficits or cancer

Treatment strategies

Following these views, introduce treatment strategies to improve the swallow and evaluate their benefit using the videofluoroscopy. Examples of these strategies include the following (see Chapters 7 and 9 for further details):

◆ Postures, such as chin tuck, head turn
◆ Sensory procedures, such as thermo-tactile stimulation, enhancing taste and texture, increasing bolus size
◆ Manoeuvres, for example supraglottic, effortful swallow
◆ Diet changes such as thickened fluids, smooth textures

Indicators for oesophageal stage examination

Groher and Crary (1997) suggest that, unless contraindicated, the oesophagus be examined. This is particularly important where the oral and pharyngeal stages are functioning adequately and there is an indication that there may be an oesophageal deficit. In the United Kingdom, radiologists have responsibility for making the decision as to whether or not to examine the oesophagus. It may be beneficial to discuss the value of this with them on an individual client basis.

Criteria for abandoning a videofluoroscopy

There is a wide discrepancy in practice over when to discontinue the procedure. 'The speech and language therapist will normally take responsibility for ... decision making in conjunction with the radiologist' (Guidelines for Radiological Imaging, RCSLT, 1999). Logemann (1998) suggests that laryngeal penetration and a small quantity of well-tolerated aspiration or pharyngeal residue are not reasons to stop, unless 10 per cent of every bolus is aspirated. However, airway obstruction, total absence of airway protection, laryngospasm and tracheo-oesophageal fistula are indicators to cease (Palmer *et al*, 1993).

If aspiration of barium has occurred, discuss with the radiologist how they suggest it be managed, as barium can set solid in the lungs. It may be appropriate to perform a chest X-ray. If the client is an inpatient, to prevent pulmonary complications, they may require physiotherapy to their chest on return to the ward. The speech and language therapist will inform the referring physician, nursing staff and physiotherapist of these results so that appropriate care is undertaken. If the client is an outpatient and is mobile, and the radiologist does not feel chest physiotherapy is indicated, explain the warning signs of a chest infection to the client and their carer and inform their family doctor immediately by telephone.

Report writing

Indicate the symptoms (residue, penetration and aspiration) and their physiological and/or anatomical causes. Treatment is directed at the physiological or anatomical cause of the symptoms, such as aspiration or residue. Next, describe the effects of the therapy strategies and make recommendations regarding feeding strategies and the method of nutritional intake (see Chapters 7 and 9). Remember to consider the client and carer's wishes regarding diet modification. Recommend therapy if appropriate, and suggest whether re-evaluation or further referral on to other professionals, such as a consultant gastroenterologist, will be indicated.

Mendelsohn (1994) describes a modified barium swallow (MBS) database, as 'every centre that caries out the MBS exam is a storehouse of useful clinical and radiological information'. He states that 'this project utilises a standardised clinical and radiological data form, which provides a consistent approach to the reporting of the MBS results'. 'The computer novice' can use it and it is menu-driven.

Some additional practical considerations

- We have found it helpful to devise and offer an information leaflet informing the client and carer about the nature of the procedure before they arrive.

- In order for the client to attend the videofluoroscopy, they may have had to wait for transport or porters, to and within the hospital, resulting in fatigue.

- The client's positioning for the procedure may be difficult owing to the nature of the X-ray equipment, and may not reflect how the client would eat or drink in their own environment.

- The examination is only a snapshot in time. The client's swallowing function may be variable, and the problem they described in the case history may not occur during the procedure. It is not representative of a meal.

- The doctor's instructions may affect the speed of the triggering of swallow: for example, 'Hold it, hold it ... and now swallow.'

- The taste, and to some extent the texture, of the radio-opaque materials is unlike any normal food or drink, and this may influence the swallow.

- The procedure potentially involves many professionals' time, and is therefore costly.

FIBRE-OPTIC ENDOSCOPIC EVALUATION OF SWALLOWING SAFETY (FEESS)

Purpose

This relatively quick and low-cost investigation assesses the pharyngeal stage of the swallow. Langmore first described it in 1988. An ear, nose and throat (ENT) surgeon and a speech and language therapist perform it. The clinician should have specialist training in its use. One of its advantages is that it can detect aspiration and the safety of oral feeding where the client's mobility precludes a videofluoroscopy. The equipment required is a 3.5mm diameter nasendoscope, a light source for the scope, a TV monitor and a videocamera with a recorder. The videotape optimises clinical use as it permits immediate client feedback and facilitates interpretation. Unlike videofluoroscopy, it allows not only assessment and regular reassessment but also the opportunity to use normal food and drink without exposure to radiation.

Candidates

FEESS can be used at the bedside or in an outpatients department, such as ENT. It can be performed on clients in intensive care units; on those who are unable to leave the ward, and when a tracheostomy is present. It is useful particularly when a prompt decision is required, for instance when a client is facing immediate discharge and videofluoroscopy is not available. It is not suitable for clients who are agitated, have a movement disorder (such as chorea or dyskinesia), small nasal passage, bleeding disorder, history of fainting or acute cardiac problems, which predispose them to bradycardia (slow heart rhythm).

Potential complications

Adverse reactions include discomfort; bleeding of the nasal mucosa; allergic reaction to the nasal anaesthetic spray and compromised afferent input to the swallow mechanism; laryngospasm (a strong aversive behaviour where mechanical stimulation of the laryngeal structures results in vocal fold adductor spasm which can lead to respiratory arrest), or a vasovagal response (the 'flight or fight' response which can result in fainting). Therefore FEESS should only be performed within an appropriate medical setting with access to medical and nursing staff, in case any unforeseen emergency occurs.

Procedure

The nasendoscope is passed via the nose by the ENT surgeon, with the tip positioned slightly lower than the uvula (see Figure 4.1). In our experience, most clients require some nasal local anaesthesia. Langmore suggests this is best given via the end of a cotton applicator. The client waits for approximately five minutes for the anaesthetic to take effect. Its action lasts for around 45 minutes. Asking the

Figure 4.1
Placement of flexible fibre-optic nasendoscope to just above the epiglottis for a FEESS

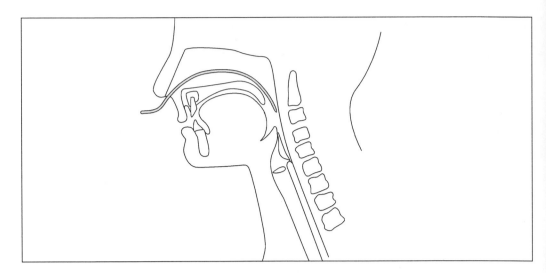

client to perform various speech, non-speech and swallowing tasks permits the assessment of the anatomy and physiology of the velum, oropharynx, hypopharynx and larynx. Swallowing is assessed by presenting food and fluid dyed with green food colouring. Green has been found to show up well in the oropharynx and larynx.

FEESS protocol (based on Langmore & Murray, 1999)

Speech and non-speech tasks

Velopharyngeal closure

◆ Phonate /a, i, m/ 'puh'.

◆ Swallow.

Hypopharynx

◆ Is it symmetrical at rest?

Vocal fold assessment

◆ Phonate on /i/ to assess adduction.

◆ Sniff to assess abduction.

◆ Breath hold to assess if the vocal folds adduct fully. Langmore and Logemann (1991) suggest that, if a client cannot achieve rapid and complete glottic closure and sustain it for a minimum of three seconds, the airway protection for swallowing will be compromised. Breath holding can be used as part of a supraglottic swallow (see Chapter 7).

◆ Cough to assess strength of glottal closure to command (see Chapter 7).

Swallowing tasks

Swallowing secretions/saliva

◆ Place two drops of food colour on the tongue; as this mixes with saliva and falls into the hypopharynx, observe flow, pooling and so on in lateral channels and in the laryngeal vestibule.

◆ Note the amount of pooling of saliva or secretions.

Swallowing food and liquid: *guidelines for assessment*

◆ Increase amount with each presentation unless aspiration occurs.

◆ Discontinue any consistency level or amount if aspiration occurs twice on the same consistency level.

◆ The order of consistencies will vary, depending on the client's needs.

◆ Try therapeutic manoeuvres such as head turn, chin tuck, supraglottic swallow (see Chapter 7) at appropriate points in the assessment, and evaluate their effectiveness.

◆ Use FEESS viewed on TV monitor for visual feedback when teaching the above therapeutic manoeuvres.

Swallowing coloured food and liquid: *consistencies to be assessed*

◆ Ice chips: begin with this consistency if the client is nil-by-mouth at present and appears to be at high risk of aspiration.

◆ Thin liquid such as milk: 5ml given via a teaspoon, working up to consecutive sips via a straw.

◆ Thick liquid such as thickened squash or juice: 5ml given via a teaspoon, working up to consecutive sips via a straw.

◆ Semi-solid such as mousse or yogurt: 5ml, 10ml, 15ml on a teaspoon or larger spoon.

◆ Solid such as biscuit or sandwich: allow client to take a bite.

Sensory assessment

◆ If sensation of the pharynx and/or larynx is thought to be reduced, sensation is tested by lightly touching (a) the posterior pharyngeal wall, (b) the mid base of the tongue, (c) epiglottis (normally this is very sensitive, and stimulating this area will elicit a response), (d) the aryepiglottic folds, and (e) the arytenoids.

Once the assessment is complete, remove the scope.

Report writing

◆ Comment on any structural abnormalities.

◆ Note pharyngeal sensation.

◆ Note the location of any pooled saliva.

◆ Describe airway protection as indicated by vocal fold function.

◆ Note any delay in triggering of the swallow reflex.

◆ Note the location of any pooled food or drink and the client's response to it.

◆ Note any laryngeal penetration or aspiration and the client's response to it.

◆ Suggest whether the client is safe to commence or increase oral intake and, if so, what consistencies and textures are recommended, and whether any therapeutic manoeuvres are to be used.

Clinical limitations

Groher and Crary (1997) suggest the results may be misinterpreted and may not be representative of the client's swallow owing to the presence of the nasendoscope. As the scope offers a limited view only, there is no information regarding potential deficits in the oral or oesophageal stages.

CERVICAL AUSCULTATION

Purpose

Cervical auscultation is a non-invasive method of evaluating the pharyngeal swallow, and can be used to aid the accuracy of the clinical dysphagia examination. Cichero (1996) says that it provides 'a portable, cost-effective and non-invasive assessment'. It utilises a stethoscope to listen to the breathing and swallowing sounds heard at the level of the laryngopharynx. Hamlet *et al* (1992) suggest that there are three physiological causes of the swallowing sounds, though this remains controversial: (a) laryngeal elevation and bolus flow through the pharynx, (b) flow through the hypopharynx and movement through the cricopharyngeal sphincter, and (c) laryngeal descent post-swallow.

Stroud (1999) suggests practising first by listening to the breathing and swallowing sounds of unimpaired individuals using water, a cube of chocolate or a fruit pastille before using the technique to assess clients with swallowing disorders. The sounds of a disordered swallow are 'less sharp or even bubbly if aspiration has occurred' (Hamlet et al, 1990). Advantages of this method are that it is cheap, highly portable, quick and repeatable. Nurses are used to using stethoscopes and they may find the technique helpful for identifying when the swallow has occurred.

Candidates

Cervical auscultation can be used on all clients, including those with tracheostomies, COPD and those in long-term care. The presence of a stethoscope held against the neck may affect the swallow. This technique is being used more frequently but has limitations, as further research is required to clarify the physiological causes of swallowing sounds.

Procedure (from Stroud, 1999)

First, wear the stethoscope with the ear pieces facing forward, following the direction of the external ear canal. At the opposite end, twisting the round bell can change the frequencies of sounds heard. The concave bell side enables low frequency breath sounds to be heard. The flat diaphragm is best for listening to swallow bursts. First, tap the bell to ensure it is 'turned on'; if it is not, turn it until it is. Next, place the bell on the lateral aspect of the neck in the region of the larynx, at the junction of the cricoid cartilage and trachea (see Figure 4.2). Listen for normal breath sounds as a baseline for that individual. Adjust the placement until the inspiration and exhalation of the cervical breath sounds are easily heard. These are usually hollow or 'tubular' when compared to the breath sounds heard when listening to the lungs. If they are noisy, ask the individual to cough and clear. The aim is to hear soft respiration.

To listen for the swallow sounds, turn the bell and tap the diaphragm to ensure it is 'on'. Ask the individual to perform a dry swallow of their saliva, then to drink water followed by thickened fluid, and finally to perform these while self-feeding, if appropriate. Listen for the swallow–breath pattern (Selley et al, 1994); see Figure

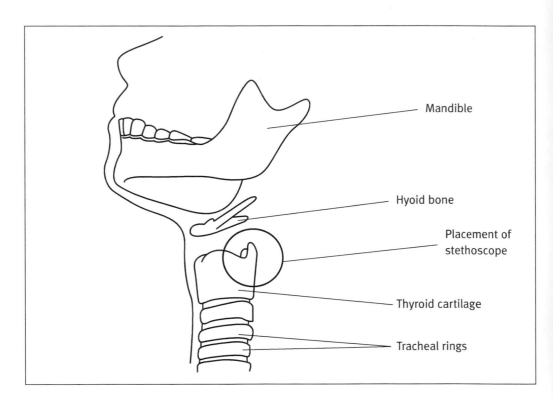

Figure 4.2
Placement of the stethoscope for cervical auscultation

4.3, which is characterised by inhalation, exhalation, apnoea, two swallow bursts or clicks as the vocal folds fully close, followed by an expiratory burst.

Zenner *et al* (1995) said that 'the pharyngeal phase was considered normal if the pharyngeal swallow occurred promptly after oral transit, an apneic period occurred during the swallow, an exhalation occurred directly after the swallow, and if clear breath sounds were heard after the swallow'.

Once the clinician learns to identify normal breath sounds, one can develop skills in recognising abnormal breathing and swallowing sounds. With a client, listen for the following:

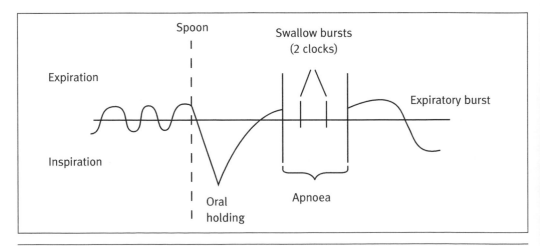

Figure 4.3
The swallow–breathing pattern

- Premature spillage of the bolus into the pharynx before the swallow is triggered.
- The two clicks of the swallow reflex – are they present or absent?
- The breath out – is it present or absent, clean or not clean sounding?
- A possible clearing swallow may be heard – is it present or absent?
- Sounds that equate with pooling or penetration, such as wet breath sounds or gurgling.

Finally, repeat, listening to the other side. Note if there is any asymmetry of pooling. Stroud suggests that water be given if the clinician feels the swallow is sufficiently safe, as clearer sounds will be heard.

Zenner *et al* (1995) go on to state that 'Impairment of the pharyngeal swallow was suspected if deviation from any of these events occurred. Tracheal aspiration was suspected when the flushing sound of material (usually liquids, similar to the sound of water running down a drain pipe) was heard prior to the initiation of the pharyngeal swallow or when wet breath sounds, stridor, coughing, throat clearing or voice distortion were heard after the swallow.' They found that 'the respiratory pattern of adults with dysphagia was different from non-impaired adults'. It is 'more variable, swallow apnoea is less consistent, and inspiration occurs more often after the swallow'.

Report writing

Stroud (1999) suggests the following notation, 'on auscultation there was evidence of the following . . .'. This may include observations such as 'bubbling heard before the bolus was given', 'no swallow reflex heard', 'liquid heard in the pharynx post swallow', 'breath sounds were not clear after the swallow', 'stridor or harsh or laboured breathing post swallow'. Recommendations are made about whether oral feeding and nutrition are safe and strategies to be implemented (see Chapter 9).

PULSE OXIMETRY

Procedure

A pulse oximeter is a device that clips on to the finger, toe or earlobe and uses red and infrared light to measure the arterial oxygen saturation of the blood. Sherman *et al* (1999) report that the technique may improve the accuracy of the bedside swallowing assessment, thereby facilitating evaluation and treatment. In this study, pulse oximetry was used with videofluoroscopy. It demonstrated that clients who exhibited aspiration or penetration without clearing the bolus, had a significant decline in oxygen saturation compared with those patients for whom the bolus penetrated but cleared, or in whom no penetration was observed. The oxygen saturation of the blood is measured in percentages. A baseline measurement is taken before assessing swallowing on fluids and foods.

Candidates

This portable non-invasive technique allows clients to be seen in a familiar setting. It permits continuous monitoring, which means it can be used for the duration of an assessment or a meal. Sherman's study showed that clients with a baseline saturation of 92 per cent had a greater decline in their saturations if they aspirated than those with a baseline saturation of 95–100 per cent.

SCINTIGRAPHY

This is a specialised investigation conducted by a radiologist specialising in nuclear medicine (ASHA, 1999a). It is an imaging technique that involves radionuclide scanning using a gamma camera during and after ingestion of a radioactive bolus. It can quantify the amount of radioactive tracer present in any region of interest, such as the pharynx (quantifying the pharyngeal transit time, pooling and the number of swallows needed to clear the pharynx), oesophagus (oesophageal transit time) and lungs (indicating the quantity of aspiration). The client who aspirates can be rescanned hours after the bolus was ingested to view the ability of the lungs to clear aspirated material. It is useful in determining whether aspiration has occurred due to reflux of the gastric contents. The speech and language therapist's role is to participate in the selection and referral of clients; help with their positioning and guide the use of swallowing manoeuvres, and contribute to the interpretation of the results and written report, particularly in the formulation of a treatment plan.

Currently, this technique is rarely employed in the United Kingdom. With further research, it may be possible, using it in combination with videofluoroscopy, to identify what is significant aspiration in populations at risk (Brown & Sonies, 1997).

ELECTROMYOGRAPHY AND SURFACE ELECTROMYOGRAPHY (SEMG)

Electromyography is the method of recording electrical activity of a muscle or a group of muscles during behaviours such as swallowing. Mainly used in research, it provides information on the onset and offset of muscle activity and the frequency of firing of motor neurones, and gives an indication of muscle strength. Bipolar, hooked-wire electrodes are inserted through the skin into the pharyngeal constrictor and the thyroarytenoid muscles. Topical anaesthetic may be required.

Surface electromyography is the recording of muscle activity obtained through electrodes applied to the skin, and thus no anaesthetic is needed. It can be used to provide biofeedback by converting the muscle activity in the laryngeal region, recorded in an auditory and/or visual display, using a small, hand-held, portable device. It is an adjunct to therapy. Crary (1995) describes its usefulness. He demonstrates improvements in swallow function and a decrease in the influence of functional decompensations (that is, when the voluntary or involuntary compensatory activities interfere with, rather than enhance, swallowing function).

SEMG biofeedback facilitates 'strength training' in manoeuvres such as Mendelsohn or super–supraglottic swallows and the coordination of sustained muscle contractions (see Chapter 7). The SEMG device is lent to the client after it has been pre-programmed by the clinician with a tailor-made hierarchy of 'strength training' tasks. By downloading and analysing the data stored in the SEMG device during the client's practice, the clinician, with the client, can review the client's accuracy in the tasks and overall progress. Depending on the results, the therapy programme can then be modified to meet the client's goal.

ULTRASOUND IMAGING

This non-invasive study using high-frequency sound waves has been found helpful in the evaluation of the soft tissues. It can be used to assess the oral stage, particularly tongue movement, but cannot be used for the pharyngeal or oesophageal stages owing to the inability of ultrasound to travel through the bones of the cervical spine or air. This technique cannot determine aspiration directly. The transducer is held against the skin of the underside of the chin to view the motion of the tongue and bolus, which is contained, transported and altered by tongue–palate control. The quality of the images and their interpretation relies largely on the skill of the ultrasonographer. As it does not involve the risks of radiation exposure it can be repeated at regular intervals and for extended durations without harm (see Perlman & Schulze-Delrieu, 1997).

MANOMETRY

This uses apparatus that measures pressure changes in the pharynx, cricopharyngeus and oesophagus. It is useful in the identification of disorders of motility. It does not offer information about aspiration. However, it can be combined with videofluoroscopy 'to accurately evaluate and diagnose dysphagia and aspiration' (Blitzer, 1990). Currently, we believe that it is used only occasionally with adults with neurogenic dysphagia in the United Kingdom, and it is more commonly used for assessing the pharyngo-oesophageal segment opening of those clients who have undergone head and neck surgery.

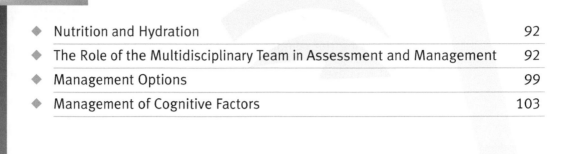

Chapter 5: General Issues in Management

NUTRITION AND HYDRATION

As stated in Chapter 3, the aim of performing a swallowing assessment is to ensure that the client can protect their airway safely, and meet their nutrition and hydration requirements. The clinician may wish to consider whether the client is able to safely commence, resume or increase their oral intake. Issues related to the key factors in predicting the complications of aspiration pneumonia are examined in Chapters 2 and 3. These include medical diagnosis – duration of disease, duration of dysphagia, progression; level of alertness; immune status; ability to mobilise; oral hygiene; presence of malnutrition and pulmonary clearance. Only a multidisciplinary team approach will reduce the risk of aspiration, malnutrition and dehydration.

Preventing dehydration is paramount when clients are unable to drink sufficient volumes. Schmidt *et al* (1994) demonstrate that evidence of aspiration on videofluoroscopy predicts pneumonia and death, but not dehydration following stroke. Therefore regular monitoring of the client's fluid intake using fluid balance charts and serum electrolytes from blood tests may be helpful to prevent dehydration (see Chapter 9).

Up to 16 per cent of clients admitted to hospital with a stroke exhibit signs of protein energy malnutrition (Axelsson et al, 1988). In other client groups this is associated with reduced stamina and life expectancy; increased susceptibility to infection; increased likelihood of pressure sores; reduced physical recovery and wound healing, and increased risk of anxiety and depression (RCSLT, 1998a). The early identification, documentation and intervention of malnutrition can improve outcome and reduce length of hospital stay (Robinson *et al*, 1987). Therefore management of dysphagia is cost-effective compared with admission to hospital for pneumonia.

THE ROLE OF THE MULTIDISCIPLINARY TEAM IN ASSESSMENT AND MANAGEMENT

Members of the multidisciplinary team

The team members will vary according to the clients' needs, the environment they live in and local policies. They include the following:

- The client, their family and carers
- Doctors: hospital – for example ENT surgeons, gastroenterologists, neurologists, radiologists; community – for example family doctors
- Hospital and community nurses
- Speech and language therapy staff
- Physiotherapy staff
- Occupational therapy staff
- Dietetic staff
- Catering staff
- Pharmacy staff
- Clinical psychology staff

The client's wishes

'The subject of feeding is an emotive issue' for the client and their family and carers (Kennedy, 1992). Sometimes, regardless of the risks explained to the client by the team, the client chooses to continue with oral food and fluid for quality of life and pleasure. In this situation it is important to document the fact that the risks of airway obstruction and pulmonary infection have been explained and discussed with the client and that they understand the implications of the risk of continuing eating and/or drinking (see Chapters 10 and 12). In other situations, the client may report that, owing to the severity of the dysphagia and fear of aspirating, oral intake brings no enjoyment and they would prefer not to be encouraged to eat or drink. In our experience, some clients have felt obliged to continue with oral intake because of the benefits perceived by the team, as oral intake is generally considered best where possible.

Responsibility of care of dysphagia

The overall responsibility for the management of the client's dysphagia rests with the client's medical practitioner. However, Kennedy (1992) states the 'decision regarding the management of the patient should not be the responsibility of one professional healthcare group alone. Instead, the multidisciplinary team should reach a joint decision regarding future management based on such factors as assessment findings, medical condition, and not least, the wishes of the patient and/or family ... If decisions regarding proposed management are not made in conjunction with all relevant personnel, it is likely that professional groups may become antagonistic and estranged, neither of which is conducive to good patient care.' Despite this recommendation, 'It remains the case that speech and language therapists are frequently asked to make recommendations about feeding after a single bedside assessment' (Kennedy *et al*, 1993).

In 'Collaborative Practice in Dysphagia' guidelines designed to promote multidisciplinary team working (RCSLT, 1995), the following are proposed:

◆ The development of coordinated assessment protocols

◆ The setting and recording of joint goals to ensure timely intervention that avoids duplication of effort

◆ Joint treatment plans with written documentation in line with local policies

◆ Fostering multidisciplinary audit of practice

◆ Adopting a common approach to the involvement of the patients, relatives and carers

The role of speech and language therapy staff (from RCSLT, 1995 and ASHA, 1999b)

◆ To assess oral motor structure and function – that is, does the patient have teeth, candida and so on?

◆ To assess the efficiency and safety of the swallow.

◆ To implement objective assessments when indicated (for example, videofluoroscopy).

◆ To determine safe feeding regimens and food consistencies.

◆ To identify and communicate the risk factors to the client, family and team members.

◆ To advise the client, their family, carers and nursing staff regarding management strategies.

◆ To monitor and to check whether the regimen is carried out, for example on the ward, in the home environment or by participation in outpatient clinics.

- To provide appropriate education and training for a range of professional staff, such as nurses and junior hospital doctors, to recognise dysphagia, the prognosis, possible complications and the client's needs in terms of food textures and fluid consistencies.

- To ensure safety, dignity, psychological and physical well-being of the client.

- To ensure that catering staff receive information and training to enable them to appreciate the importance of specific food consistencies, and to produce these with the required nutritional supplement as advised by the dietitian.

- To be an advocate for the client.

- To be sensitive to the client's economic, educational and employment background and cultural beliefs.

- To establish links with appropriate members of the MDT and to facilitate team communication.

- To document the activity of the team.

- To maintain the team's focus.

Further information on legal and professional issues is contained in Chapter 10.

The role of physiotherapy staff

The physiotherapists' contribution involves the following:

- Positioning the client; and recommendations and use of appropriate seating and other postural support to facilitate safe and effective feeding and swallowing (see Chapter 3)

- Positioning of any assistant who helps with meals to minimise their fatigue and strain

- Preparation of the client for feeding by ensuring tone is as normal as possible and the chest is clear

- Maintenance of the client's respiratory system

- The use of suction and humidification

- Monitoring of the client's chest

The role of occupational therapy staff

'Collaborative Practice in Dysphagia' (RCSLT, 1995) suggests that the occupational therapist considers the impact of physical, environmental, social and behavioural factors in the assessment and management of clients with dysphagia. This may involve:

◆ Joint working to facilitate positioning (see Chapter 3), which may involve use of appropriate seating

◆ Facilitating independence through positioning or the use of adaptive equipment

◆ Assessing the impact of cognitive, perceptual and behavioural impairments and other social factors with the clinical psychologist and facilitating effective management

The role of nursing staff

The United Kingdom Central Council for Nursing, Midwifery and Health Visiting (1997) states that 'nurses have a clear responsibility for ensuring the nutritional needs of patients ... nurses have an implicit responsibility for ensuring that patients are fed ... Nurses may delegate the task of feeding patients, for example to unregistered practitioners, but ... overall responsibility remains with the registered nurse'. The benefit of assisting clients with feeding is that 'It provides an opportunity to observe and monitor aspects of a patient's progress, both psychological and physical. Without this involvement, judgements about a patient will be made with incomplete information.'

Nurses assist clients with the mixing of thickening agents, selecting appropriate consistencies from menus, and ordering supplements as recommended by the speech and language therapist and dietitian. In hospitals, they ensure that appropriate signs are placed above the clients' beds, such as those indicating nil-by-mouth or thickened fluids only, in collaboration with the recommendations of the team. They help the client and carers with keeping food and fluid intake charts.

In most settings it is the role of the nurse to pass a nasogastric tube and to confirm it is sited in the stomach rather than the lungs. This is achieved by using a syringe to withdraw a small amount of the stomach contents up the tube and then checking its acidity on litmus paper. This is commonly used in combination with a stethoscope to listen for air syringed into the tube entering the stomach. Clients with swallowing disorders may experience difficulty with the passing of a nasogastric tube. This is because the larynx may not elevate fully on attempts to swallow the tube down, resulting in failure of the opening of the cricopharyngeal sphincter. In such cases, it may be necessary to pass the tube under x-ray guidance, confirming its position in the stomach. Some multidisciplinary teams may have clinical nurse specialists who are particularly skilled at passing nasogastric tubes. They may provide counselling pre- and post-insertion of gastrostomy tubes to the client and their carers as well as teaching them how to use the equipment.

The role of dietetic staff

Part of the dietitian's role is to calculate the nutritional requirements of clients and participate in selecting the route(s) of administration (see Chapter 9). They monitor the client's intake against their requirements using food and feed record charts, biochemistry, fluid input and output charts, visual observation and the client's weight. From this, they modify intake and advise on a change in the route of administration, if required. They work closely with the nursing staff, carers, catering, pharmacy and medical staff (see Chapter 9). For those clients who are discharged home on a feed, they arrange for the appropriate feed and pump to be delivered to the client's home environment.

The role of pharmacy staff

Pharmacists advise on types of medication, doses and how best to administer them. For clients who are at risk of aspiration on tablets and fluids, many medications can be given in liquid (elixir) or dispersible form. Others may be injectable or administered under the tongue (sublingually), percutaneously (using patches) or per rectum. Those that are in liquid, dispersible or crushable form can be mixed with thickening powder or food, if required (see Chapter 7). Slow release or enteric-coated tablets should not be crushed, as this action will destroy the formulation leading to premature absorption and possible toxicity. The same may apply to some capsules, so the pharmacist is able to check with the manufacturers and advises whether and how the contents may be administered. Crushing tablets and pouring enteric-coated granules from capsules can lead to the blocking of feeding tubes (Shulman, 1997).

Pharmacists can suggest medications to help reflux; to thin secretions; to supplement or decrease salivary flow, and to provide external lubrication and muscle relaxants (for example for cricopharyngeal spasms and hiccups). They can provide information about medications that adversely affect the swallow mechanism (see Chapter 3), and on dyes for checking leaks in tubes. Pharmacists advise on prokinetic agents (such as metaclopramide or cisapride), which increase bowel motility, thereby increasing absorption and reducing the likelihood of aspiration of the nasogastric or percutaneous gastrostomy feed. Conversely, they can identify drugs such as morphine, which can decrease gastric motility, thus adversely affecting absorption. They advise on the timing of drugs in relation to food and enteral feeds (see Chapter 9). For instance, potential drug–enteral feed interactions include phenytoin, warfarin and antacids. Medications for the management of Parkinson's disease, myasthenia gravis and multiple sclerosis may have a positive impact on the client's swallowing mechanism if administered at the appropriate time before eating and drinking. Fonda *et al* (1995) describe how a 72-year-old man with a nine-year history of Parkinson's disease had lost 30kg in weight over an 18-month period. When his anti-Parkinsonian medication was taken one hour before mealtimes, his blood levels of the medication peaked during the meal. He reported that he felt his swallowing had improved, and this was supported by videofluoroscopy assessment. Also this was borne out by his weight gain.

Staff education and training

The speech and language therapist plays a key role in multidisciplinary training to facilitate staff awareness and understanding of dysphagia and its complications. The Scottish Intercollegiate Guidelines Network (1997) suggests that topics may include the client's needs with regard to food texture, safety, dignity, psychological and physical well-being. It also states that catering staff require 'information and training to enable them to appreciate the importance of specific food consistencies and to prepare appropriate meals or food items, with any necessary nutritional supplementation advised by a dietitian'. See also Chapter 13.

Specialist clinics

Specialist swallowing clinics are becoming more common in the United Kingdom. Neurologists, ENT surgeons or consultant radiologists may run these with speech and language therapists, dietitians and nurses. These facilitate the appropriate assessment, management and monitoring of dysphagia, and lead to the possibility of multidisciplinary audit and research. Torrance (1996) argues that multidisciplinary gastrostomy clinics allow clients to be reviewed by the same team of professionals each time, thus providing them and the professionals with a structured approach and support. It allows the client 'to progress at the most beneficial and safest rate', the goal being returning 'to oral intake whenever possible and ensuring nutritional stability'. She states that 'the gastrostomy clinic is also extremely helpful in monitoring patients with Motor Neurone Disease'. The final advantage of such a clinic is to offer the client a point of contact in the hospital to monitor the gastrostomy site and tube, thus avoiding complications. A gastrostomy tube can remain in place for up to two years before it requires changing.

MANAGEMENT OPTIONS

Following the outcome of the MDT's decision, and depending on the diagnosis, prognosis, severity of the dysphagia, the client's motivation, interest, cognitive skills and ability to follow directions, respiratory function and availability of caregiver support, the clinician will decide on the most appropriate form of management. Crary, Logemann and Kennedy all offer different ways of approaching management. These three approaches will be expanded on, to aid clinical practice: (a) medical, surgical and behavioural management, (b) direct or indirect therapy, and (c) active therapy or advice only.

Medical, surgical and behavioural management

Crary (from Groher & Crary, 1997) states that the treatment options are medical, surgical or behavioural (see Chapters 7, 8 and 9). Medical options include dietary modifications such as regulating nutrition and hydration, special diets and alternative sources of nutrition and hydration. Part of this approach is the pharmacological management (see the role of pharmacy staff, above). Surgical options may be those that improve glottal closure (for example, phonosurgery); protect the airway (for example, tracheostomy tubes or laryngectomy), or increase the opening of the cricopharyngeal sphincter (for example, dilation, myotomy or injecting Botulinum toxin). In our experience, the reduced opening of the cricopharyngeal sphincter is rare without other physiological symptoms (see Chapter 7). Behavioural therapies include modifying the following: the food, the feeding activity, the patient, the mechanism and the swallow. Modifying the food involves looking at viscosity, volume, temperature, lubricity and aesthetics. Modifying the feeding activity requires thinking about the timing of meals, such as not eating when fatigued after physiotherapy rehabilitation, lubricating the oropharynx with a sip of drink before eating, supplying equipment such as non-slip mats and adapted utensils to facilitate independent feeding and oral hygiene after meals. Modifying the client's behaviour may involve prompting them to slow down their rate of self-feeding, using a chin down position when swallowing and remaining upright for 30 minutes after a meal to prevent reflux. The mechanism itself can be modified by offering exercises including strengthening, range of motion, control and coordination, for example of chewing, breathing and swallowing. Finally, the swallow can be modified by using instrumental feedback (such as from videofluoroscopy, FEESS or SEMG), and from teaching techniques such as an effortful or supraglottic swallow.

The combination of treatment options utilised will depend on consideration of the following:

- The timing of the treatment – is the client recovering, stable or fluctuating?
- The types of treatment – are they preventative or prophylactic, passive or active, client- or environment-centred?
- Follow-up issues – will the client be willing and able to participate, and is it necessary to repeat any of the investigations?

Direct or indirect therapy

Direct therapy

According to Logemann (1998), this term refers to working directly on swallowing. This means using food and/or drink and asking the client to swallow while following specific instructions (for head turn and/or supraglottic swallow, for example: see Chapter 7), which are reinforced by a written cue card. The rationale for the strategies is explained and discussed with the client, who is given time to practise them without food or drink to start with. Only small sips or mouthfuls are offered for the practice swallows, to reassure the client that the bolus will not obstruct the airway. The client is encouraged not to inhibit coughing because they may feel 'it is a sign of failure to swallow correctly. Instead, they should be positively reinforced for coughing as needed'.

Indirect therapy

This refers to exercises to improve motor control without swallowing food or drink. It may involve practising swallowing saliva. It is commonly used where clients aspirate on all food and drink and are unsafe for any oral intake. Logemann (1998) advises that 'It is of no help to place a patient in a situation where he or she is continuously aspirating with no hope of deterring material from entering the airway during the swallowing regimen.' We advocate that those clients with chest infections or severely compromised respiratory systems are not candidates for oral intake until their chest status resolves. This is because they are more likely to aspirate, as it is more difficult to coordinate respiration and swallowing in these conditions. Chest status can be used as a baseline from which to compare the progress and outcome, to judge the safety of the swallow. This cannot be used if a chest infection exists from the outset. Finally, these clients are likely to feel unwell and may not be interested in eating or drinking. Instead, clients with a chest infection may benefit from indirect therapy if they are medically stable and motivated, and the fatiguing effect of such exercises is limited.

Logemann goes on to suggest that only videofluoroscopy can provide the necessary information to decide whether a client is a candidate for direct or indirect therapy. In our experience, in the United Kingdom, many clients do not have access to videofluoroscopy, and so a (tentative) hypothesis for the impairment of the swallow physiology may be made by observation during the clinical evaluation, from which adequate management decisions may be made. The hypothesis can be modified, in line with the client's ability to change, at any time during assessment and management.

Active therapy or advice only to clients and carers

Kennedy (1992) suggests that 'active therapy is directed towards improving the swallow pattern and minimising the risk of aspiration'. This is what Logemann calls direct therapy. Kennedy suggests an alternative to indirect therapy – that is, advice to clients and carers only. This aims to minimise the risk of aspiration on oral intake and to increase patient comfort. It is suitable for clients for whom an active and more aggressive therapeutic approach is inappropriate, such as those in the end stages of terminal or progressive illness, those with significant cognitive deficits or the very frail elderly. The client may be offered advice regarding positioning, modification of dietary consistencies and strategies to optimise the environment to facilitate safer eating and drinking. This advice is generally given in collaboration with the multidisciplinary team, notably physiotherapy, dietetic and occupational therapy staff. The proposed type of intervention is always discussed with the medical team and their agreement sought before it is commenced. The multidisciplinary team is informed of the medical agreement and any future changes in the approach. Kennedy says, 'This liaison between relevant professions is necessary to confirm that safe feeding practices are implemented thus ensuring the patient's well-being.'

Documentation and reporting

The clinician writes in the speech and language therapy notes within 24 hours of the event, whether it be assessment, advice, management or the fact that the client is unavailable. The consistencies and volumes given are documented. 'A written, individualised care plan will be placed in the nursing notes or at the bedside for inpatients or given to the patient or carer in the case of outpatients [see Appendix

IV for examples]. Verbal reports will be made to medical, nursing and other appropriate staff' (Scottish Intercollegiate Guidelines Network, 1997). The medical notes are updated as appropriate, with summaries of assessment results and progress, and whether there is a proposed change in management. (See Chapter 10 for further details of legal and professional issues.)

Discharge

Discharge planning occurs continually throughout assessment and management. These plans depend on factors such as severity, diagnosis and outcome. They are made in agreement with the client and multidisciplinary team and are documented. The client, their carers and the team are given information on how to contact the speech and language therapy department in the future and re-refer if necessary, should the situation change. Potential reasons for discharge are listed below (Scottish Intercollegiate Guidelines Network, 1997):

◆ No abnormality detected

◆ Assessment and advice

◆ Problem resolved

◆ Modified regime established and/or present potential realised

◆ Deteriorating medically

◆ Non-compliance

◆ Transferred (including to other therapist)

◆ Failure/unable to attend

◆ Died

◆ Therapist withdrawal

MANAGEMENT OF COGNITIVE FACTORS

Many of the strategies described are simple common sense, and may be used in combination. It may be useful to read this section in combination with Chapter 9, 'Nutrition and Hydration'.

Difficulties with cognitive aspects of swallowing may occur together with neurological swallowing problems, or present in isolation. Referrals from rehabilitation and continuing care units frequently relate to longer-term behavioural swallowing problems. The aetiologies of such problems include dementia and other globally impairing disorders, and single non-dominant (normally right) hemisphere lesions. These clients may fail to meet their anticipated rehabilitation goals owing to their underlying cognitive and language problems. For example, two clients presenting with a marked lower facial weakness, one arising from a left hemisphere stroke, the other from a right hemisphere stroke, may achieve very different outcomes dependent solely on the side of the lesion. The former would normally be able to implement strategies (devised by themselves and/or the clinician) to cope with a range of textures despite the facial weakness. The latter may experience significant delay in resuming a normal oral diet.

Management strategies for a client who forgets to swallow

◆ Self-feeding is important, even if it is facilitated by another.

◆ Always wait until the client is fully alert and awake, and reduce distractions.

◆ Ensure that the client is hungry and/or thirsty. This is particularly important for those on non-oral regimes, and should be considered even if only tastes-for-pleasure are being offered. Shared management with the nutrition team is essential.

◆ Provide verbal prompt(s) to swallow.

◆ Presenting the next spoon/forkful may help elicit a swallow reflex. Alternatively, remove the spoon/fork from a client's mouth so that they can swallow.

◆ Modify the bolus to a consistency which may be more stimulating, either for all oral intake or interspersed within the meal if the client's attention begins to wane: for example, chilled bolus, sour bolus, fizzy drinks.

◆ Clients with dementia often require a larger bolus to trigger a swallow.

◆ If necessary, avoid foods which can be chewed and chewed, although the majority of clients will benefit from and need some texture to ensure kinaesthetic feedback. They may swallow normal fluids promptly since they require less preparation. If purée is indicated, ensure that it is appetising and presented so that the client can distinguish the different tastes.

Management strategies for a client who fatigues quickly

This would be an anticipated scenario for a frail, elderly, malnourished person, with a progressive neurological disorder. It may be helpful to consider the following strategies to prevent fatigue and enhance nutrition and hydration:

- Size and frequency of meals: small, frequently spaced.
- Oral versus non-oral feeding – it may be appropriate to consider supplementing oral intake with top-ups via an alternative route. This can reduce the client's feeling of being under pressure to complete all meals and drinks offered.
- Timing of oral intake within the day's structure or routine: it may be helpful to consider suitably long rest periods between oral intake, as well as other activities, such as washing, dressing, physiotherapy and seeing visitors. A formal timetable for both the client and their carers may be of benefit.
- Investigations: objective assessments of swallowing should be kept to a minimum since, not only are they fatiguing procedures, but they are, by their nature, unlikely to show the client's true skills.
- Indirect or direct management: the latter is indicated to minimise fatigue.

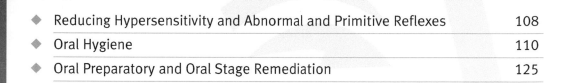

Chapter 6: Oral Stage Management

REDUCING HYPERSENSITIVITY AND ABNORMAL AND PRIMITIVE REFLEXES

Some primitive reflexes, such as rooting, may be utilised to a client's advantage. Abnormal reflexes (bite and tongue thrust) and hypersensitivity may require desensitisation to reduce them to a manageable level before further management can progress. Appropriate positioning of a client (see Figure 6.1) may be sufficient to overcome a large proportion, if not all, of these problems.

It is useful to note that it is not always necessary to inhibit a reflex before going on to the next stage – for example, starting to chew may help inhibit a bite or gag reflex. A basic desensitisation programme is provided by Kennedy (unpublished, 1992). Before commencing, reduce any background noise and distractions. Tell the client what you are going to do at each stage. For example, you say 'one, two, three' and carry out the action on three to reduce anticipation.

Start working with a gentle but firm touch, on areas of the body on which the patient is used to having contact, such as the torso, then the lower limbs, then the upper limbs. Always start at the distal points and work more proximally, backtracking if the client shows even the smallest sign of increased tone or distress.

If the patient still seems fairly intolerant of contact, but gets to the point of generally accepting some touch on the torso or limbs, it is worth considering using additional but different materials on these parts of the body, before progressing to the more

Figure 6.1
Ideal posture involves symmetry: an extended or upright trunk, upright head with chin tuck, flexion at the hips and knees, with both feet flat on the floor.

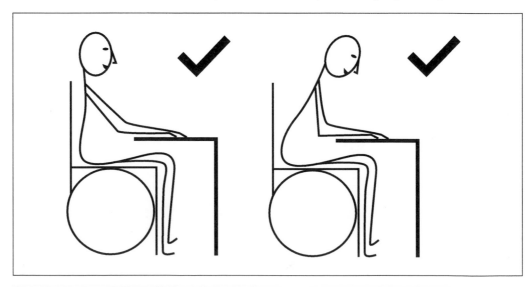

sensitive areas. Examples of types of materials are soft cotton, velvet, real sponge, cotton wool and towelling. It is always very important to apply these with gentle but firm pressure in a small, stroking action. Overly light touch can be unpleasant and tickle. It is also valuable to take time when carrying out the procedure.

Once the patient has developed tolerance to these areas, move up the back of the neck and head, coming gradually over the cranium towards the forehead and then to the cheeks and down towards the mouth. Again the actions should be carried out with gentle but firm stroking movements. Different textures can again be used here. For someone who is extremely hypersensitive, it is quite usual to notice a marked delineation in the lower half of the face, and to find that this area together with that immediately around the mouth and inside the oral cavity, are the more sensitive areas. Caution therefore needs to be taken when approaching this area.

As with all desensitisation, sometimes patients can tolerate the touch coming from their own hand, rather than someone else's. Ways of managing this are to guide the person's hand to the part of the body to which you are going to provide the stimulus, and then help them to carry out the firm stroking action.

If it is still difficult for the client to open their mouth, it is worth considering trying to elicit or facilitate more spontaneous mouth opening. This can be done through activities such as dropping some water (not ice cold) on to the lips, or wetting a large cotton bud and moistening the lips with this. Given time, the temperomandibular joint and the masseter will relax and the mouth will open, or the client will spontaneously initiate activity such as lip smacking or licking the lips.

If the client is able to tolerate the clinician facilitating lip opening, but cannot release the clenched jaw, and it seems fairly certain that this is not due to a bite reflex per se but rather to increased tone, the clinician can moisten their gloved index finger and run this along the client's gums from front to back in a slow rhythmical way. Often this will release the increased tone in the jaw, and will also noticeably relax the tongue, meaning that it goes from a retracted humped posture to coming more forward in the mouth.

When it gets to the point of introducing something to the client's mouth, such as a toothbrush, it is always helpful to let them hold the implement with the clinician guiding their hand.

Examples of desensitisation programmes are provided in Appendix IV.

ORAL HYGIENE

This section addresses the following areas:

◆ Why oral hygiene is an issue

◆ Whose role it is

◆ Saliva

◆ Mouth care problems and management techniques

◆ Good practice in mouth care

◆ Coping with reduced saliva

◆ Coping with drooling

◆ Dentures

Why oral hygiene is an issue

This section contains detailed information relating to the maintenance of good oral hygiene, to stress the importance of this area in client management. A client's ability to manage their saliva is assessed early in the clinical swallowing evaluation. The oral cavity is extremely sensitive to changes in the quality and content of its saliva. Dehydration, infection and dental problems are a small number of the potential causes of disrupted oral hygiene, and hence the client's ability to swallow their saliva.

Inadequate oral hygiene leads to:

◆ A loss of dignity

◆ Reduced and unpleasant oral sensation

◆ A coated tongue, causing reduced range of movement

◆ Increased bacteria, presenting a high risk of chest infection if this saliva is aspirated

◆ Food residue from pocketing, increasing the number of bacteria present, causing a bad taste in the mouth and reducing others' interaction with the affected person

Whose role is it?

The speech and language therapist may be involved in administering mouth care at the start of an assessment or treatment session, but responsibility rests with the nursing team as part of a client's personal hygiene. Where possible, clients should be provided with the tools to carry out their own oral hygiene (as per self-feeding).

Despite oral care being a topic of many nursing articles, there is a gulf between theory and practice in relation to nurse-administered oral hygiene. Guidelines, if they exist, tend to be informal, and may not provide sufficient guidance. In particular, there is a paucity of information regarding coping with those clients who have their own teeth, or those with oromotor problems. Definitions of mouth care may relate only to the care of dentures.

The majority of nursing staff find performing mouth care unpleasant. The task is frequently delegated:

◆ To auxiliaries, with limited or no training in techniques.
◆ To night staff. Training for permanent night staff is rarely offered, and while dentures may be soaked, those clients with their own teeth and the edentulous (those with no teeth) are frequently forgotten.
◆ To the denture-wearing nurse, who is usually viewed as the in-house expert. Staff's own dental hygiene practices appear to influence those with their clients. There is therefore a need for training in performing their own oral hygiene before they can be expected to change their client care.

Nurses may view some groups of clients as difficult to work with (for example, those with cognitive or communication impairments). These clients may be unable to alert their carers to their needs. Equipment may not be readily available or within reach. It may not be clear who is responsible for ordering mouth care equipment, or from whose budget the equipment is to be purchased.

Advice from the pharmacy, dental and medical teams is also essential to effective patient management.

Saliva

Whole saliva is a complex fluid that is produced by (a) three pairs of major salivary glands – the parotid (clear watery fluid), sublingual (predominantly serous fluid) and submandibular (predominantly mucus); (b) numerous minor salivary glands found deep in the mucosa of the upper and lower lips, the cheeks, the undersurface of the tongue, the soft palate, the dorsal surface of the tongue and the lateral parts of the hard palate behind the first premolar, and (c) fluid from the gingival crevice.

The quantity of saliva produced depends on many individual factors, such as gender, age, hydration and stress. Generally, people secrete more saliva when they are upright than when lying down (Johnson & Scott, 1993). If the volume falls outside that person's norm by 50 per cent or more (whatever the starting value), symptoms of a dry mouth will develop. Approximately one to one-and-a-half litres of saliva are produced each day. Normal healthy adults swallow their saliva approximately once or twice a minute (McCulloch *et al*, in Perlman and Schulze-Delrieu, 1997).

Functions of saliva (Kaplan & Baum, 1993)

Saliva has numerous functions, including lubrication of the tongue and lips during speech. Its other functions are given below:

1   *Dental protection.* Bacteria and plaque (see below) lower the pH within the oral cavity to acid levels that may then threaten the teeth by attacking their surface structure. Salivary proteins ensure that the saliva is supersaturated with calcium and phosphate, which are in a state of flux on the tooth surfaces, thereby creating a constant reservoir of substances to rebuild tooth structure lost by the attacking acid.

    Assuming sufficient saliva is present, it washes away acid quickly. Yet, even with adequate saliva, following only one mouthful of food or drink, it can take between 20 and 120 minutes for the mouth to return to its safe pH level (pH 6–7). In addition, the lubricating features of saliva reduce frictional wear and protect against mineral loss secondary to caries by forming a protective film on the tooth surface. The saliva produced in older age appears to have fewer protective properties.

2   *Mucosal protection.* Just as it coats the teeth, saliva affords protection to the oral mucosa against desiccation and frictional abrasion. This protection is called the mucosal pellicle. Saliva may also be involved in oral wound healing.

3   *Maintains pH.* Saliva affords protection against acid that attacks the teeth. It also neutralises residual gastric acids in the oesophagus and therefore reduces reflux. An increase in saliva produced in response to gastro-oesophageal reflux is a protective mechanism against mucosal damage.

4   *Antimicrobial action.* Saliva destroys micro-organisms and clears toxic substances. It is (a) antibacterial – the oral cavity contains flora that, although pathogenic, generally pose no mortal risk to the individual. They are likely to be present in order to prevent colonisation by other, more fatal organisms. These normal bacteria feed on salivary sugars, using them up so that no food remains for other bacteria; (b) antifungal – there is some candida albicans (see below) present in normal flora, but the quantity is controlled by an intact immune system; (c) antiviral – saliva appears to possess some neutralising effects on viruses.

5   *Digestive actions.* Saliva acts as a solvent for tastants in food; as a vehicle for delivering tastant to the taste buds; to lubricate food to assist in chewing and bolus formation; in processing food into constituents (for example, digestion of carbohydrates starts in the mouth); and as an oesophageal lubricant.

Mouth care problems and management techniques

There is disagreement as to whether the problems detailed below affect swallowing. It does appear, however, that significant dysphagia may be observed if one of these problems is superimposed on existing (normally mild) dysphagia, particularly candidiasis.

Problems related to plaque (for those with teeth)

Dental caries (tooth decay) is caused by acid destroying the tooth crowns, resulting in pain and infection.

Periodontal (gum) disease ultimately has an effect on tooth and bone structure. Plaque left untreated for as little as three days will start to break down the periodontal layer, and is therefore equally a problem in edentulous clients. Gingivitis will start to appear within 10 days. Calculus (hardened plaque) is believed to form significantly faster in tube-fed patients, therefore plaque removal is a priority.

Understanding plaque acid

The bacteria contained in the normal oral flora produce acid (see preceding section on saliva). Dental plaque serves to hold the acid in contact with the teeth. These bacteria are fed principally by sugars (for example, sucrose and glucose), either from those present in the ingested food and drink, or from the initial breakdown of this food or drink by the saliva. Plaque itself is a mixture of slime produced by the bacteria feeding on sugars. It is not water-soluble.

How speech and language therapists can contribute to the minimisation and elimination of plaque

Consider the consistencies and food types used when managing dysphagia. Elixirs of many drugs encourage caries since they contain large quantities of sugar. Suggest low sugar, non-retentive snacks, such as yogurt or cottage cheese. Soft textured foods such as bananas are often orally retentive and, since they are normally the type to contain sucrose, they pose a significant risk of bone and tooth destruction. Artificial sweeteners do not have the same effect on plaque. Carbonated drinks can decrease tooth enamel and lead to dental caries.

Fluoride reduces the susceptibility to decay. Older people may be more susceptible to root canal caries and therefore need extra fluoride. The levels of fluoride in toothpaste are normally sufficient.

For dentures see also the section on dentures later in this chapter. Glass ionomer cements that release fluoride may help to reduce caries if there are some natural teeth present.

Brushing is the only sure way to remove plaque since it is not water-soluble. The aim is to remove plaque without damaging the teeth or gums. The advocated method of brushing is 'scrub tooth brushing': this uses short, gentle, unhurried, systematic, horizontal, small strokes at the neck of the tooth (the gingival margins). Use a toothbrush with a small head (22–28mm × 10–13mm), soft–medium texture and densely packed filaments. Toothpaste is not essential, but it multiplies the mechanical effect of brushing. All toothpaste must be removed with – an aspirating toothbrush, a moist swab or suction. Toothpaste should be removed from the oral cavity since it has a drying effect.

Chlorhexidine (for example, Corsodyl) is an antiseptic liquid which is useful in controlling plaque by reducing its progress. It is available in gel or spray form for direct application to teeth and gums. Its advantages are that it need only be used once (10ml) every 12 hours. The disadvantages are that it can be used for only one month owing to adverse side effects; it has a very strong mint flavour taste; it stains teeth (this stain can be removed by a dentist); and it needs to be held in the mouth for up to one minute to have an effect.

More susceptible groups (diabetics, those with oral wounds, the immunosuppressed and those with cardiac disease) need superior mouth care.

Regular dental check-ups are important for all groups. Note: the incidence of oral cancer has been reported to be similar to that of cervical cancer. A dentist is often the first to detect it.

Candidiasis. A yeast-like pathogenic fungus, candida albicans (also called monilia) causes candidiasis. Candidiasis is the commonest infection of the mouth in the over-70s. Wearing dentures increases the candida oral population. Chronic candida is seen in 65 per cent of denture wearers (reddened, painless areas). Candida occurs normally on skin, and in the mouth (as part of the existing flora), but the onset of candidiasis implies a relaxation of the normal immune defences, not necessarily an infection of a new 'foreign' strain. Candidiasis can be of three types:

1   *Perleche*: characterised by cracking of the labial junctions. Marked by lesions on the lips and at the angles of the mouth (also known as angular chelations). Possibly related to riboflavin deficiency.

2   *Sub-acute thrush*: manifesting as flaky, loose creamy coloured plaque, covering a bright red and inflamed mucous membrane.

3   *Chronic thrush*: which manifests itself as reddened buccal mucosa, sometimes patchy, and a swollen, red, smooth-surfaced tongue. An outbreak of thrush may affect the oral, pharyngeal and oesophageal cavities.

Possible management includes the following:

◆   Antifungal treatment – *Nystatin* oral suspension (2ml held in the mouth for two minutes, to be effective, needs to be used four-hourly, for five days). It is also available in pastille form; *Ketoconazole* (200mg orally, once daily, for five days). There is a possibility of serious side effects; *Fluconazole* (150mg orally, as single dose). Unlike the others, it is absorbed from the gastrointestinal tract and therefore can be taken orally.

◆   Dentures – non-metal dentures may be soaked in Milton, or in other dilute chlorine-releasing solutions; metal dentures may be brushed with Povidine–iodine solution.

◆   Universal precautions must always be used, since candida can be transmitted by hand.

◆   Treat the underlying causes (if they exist), such as altered immune deficiency, or wait for the problem to resolve, for example if related to antibiotic use.

Ulcers

It is helpful to trace the source of ulcers if possible, and to correct the cause. There are two types:

1   White ulceration (aphthous ulceration). This is due to underlying conditions such as vitamin B12 deficiency or iron deficiency anaemia. Possible

management includes tetracycline suspension mouthwash, rinsing with 250mg for two minutes (which should then be swallowed), every six hours.

2 Bleeding or traumatic ulcers, which may be due to damaged or fractured teeth or rough tooth surfaces.

Benzydamine hydrochloride rinse or spray provides relief from oral ulceration, but occasional side effects include numbness or stinging.

Acute inflammations of oropharyngeal tissue

This includes herpes simplex. Possible management may involve oral acyclovir, 200mg, four-hourly for one week, or 400mg if the client is immunosuppressed; also chemotherapy or astringent mouthwashes.

Good practice in mouth care

There is a copious literature, much of it nursing, devoted to oral hygiene. The level of agreement between texts, and the depth of rationale given for different practices, varies enormously.

Frequency of mouth care

The frequency of mouth care appears to be a significant and more important factor than the type of agent used. Attention every four hours has only a transient and minimal effect in removing debris, while omission of care for between two and six hours significantly reduces the benefits of previously consistent care. Some texts recommend hourly mouth care (throughout the day and night), even if this requires waking the client.

Tools

Plaque is the major oral hygiene problem for clients (see above). Therefore nothing will work as well as a toothbrush, possibly aided by toothpaste if appropriate. American texts refer to aspirating toothbrushes (for example, Plak Vac, Aspir-Brush), which may be useful for the client with poor oral function, but these do not appear to be easily available in the United Kingdom. Brushing the tongue is also recommended, although dentists report that there is no evidence to support this. There appears to be an overall concern among nurses as to how much pressure to use when delivering oral care. For interdental spaces, dental floss or tape is recommended; or, if the teeth are widely spaced, strips of gauze used in the same way. Small inter-space toothbrushes may be useful.

Foam swabs are the preferred choice of nurses, but only 20 per cent of clients like this method. They are not considered effective in removing plaque. They may be useful for treating inflamed tissues, so as not to traumatise the mouth further, but there is a risk of compressing debris and plaque into the crevices and gaps of the teeth. Mouth care packs are often available, but tend to encourage one approach to mouth care, rather than taking each individual's needs into account via a complete assessment. Ideally, foam swabs should only be used for mopping up debris, using a rotating action.

For dried, quite thick and hardened secretions in the oral cavity, Groher (1984) recommends gentle but regular removal with a damp washcloth. It has also been suggested that food residue may be removed with a suction catheter, swab or washcloth. For clients whose oral mucosa has become excessively dry owing to mouth breathing, where use of a toothbrush, washcloth or foam stick causes trauma to the delicate mucosa, we suggest spreading KY jelly with a gloved finger over the tongue and palate. This may also protect the mucosa from further drying and soften dried secretions, allowing them to be removed gently.

Agents

Above all, the clinician must ensure that any agents used do not have a damaging effect, particularly on the mucosa. Ideally an agent should be alkaline (normal pH of the mouth is between 6 and 7), exert bacteriostatic effects and control plaque deposition. Agents commonly referred to in the literature are listed in Table 6.1.

Table 6.1 Mouthcare: Advantages and Disadvantage of Agents

AGENT	ADVANTAGES	DISADVANTAGES
Normal tap water	Non abrasive Acceptable to most clients	Does not reduce plaque
Tellodent pink effervescent tablets	Mild antiseptic Non-abrasive Acceptable to most clients	Does not reduce plaque
Saline Irrigation with warm solution of 0.9 per cent saline (4.5g = 1 level teaspoon per 500ml water), or sterile sachets of normal saline for the immunosuppressed	May be used to bathe crusted lips Cheap and easy to use, but it is not clear whether it is more effective than water A warm solution of saline is recommended in the management of mucositis, the serious inflammation of the mucosa due to chemotherapy or radiotherapy	
KY or clear lubricant jelly	Lubricates dry, cracked lips and oral mucosa; may prevent further loss of moisture	
Vaseline or a lanolin-based cream	Lubricates dry, cracked lips and prevents further loss of moisture	Should be avoided on lips or tongue where there is a risk of aspiration pneumonia, as oil is highly damaging to the lungs
Unsweetened tinned pineapple	Cleans the tongue with gentle brushing or chewing (pineapple chunks contain a proteolytic enzyme, ananase, that cleans the mouth)	Naturally high in sugars; oral residue can encourage plaque and caries formation
Sodium bicarbonate (1g per 100ml warm water)	Mucosolvent that reduces the viscosity of tenacious mucus Effervescent cleansing action	Not useful for long-standing or hardened debris Unpleasant taste Not well researched, and use may be time limited, to ensure that urea and electrolytes are not affected
1:1 cider and soda water	Gentle effervescent cleansing action	Exercise extreme caution with clients with dysphagia
Hydrogen peroxide (3 per cent)	Mildly antiseptic, mucosolvent, effervescent cleansing action	Unpleasant taste Potential chemical burns if not correctly diluted
Lemon and glycerine swabs		Usefulness is questionable While the glycerine is lubricating, it is also astringent The lemon stimulates saliva, so overuse may exhaust the salivary glands Low pH increases the risk of dental caries

Coping with reduced saliva

Quantities

If the quantity of saliva falls outside an individual's norm by 50 per cent or more (whatever the starting value), symptoms of a dry mouth will develop.

Reported effects of reduced saliva

All of the following potentially result in changes in taste sensation, and loss of appetite:

◆ Dry mouth
◆ Diminished volume, and thicker consistency of saliva. Accumulation of stringy mucus, which has lost its lubricating abilities. This is a very common complaint post-radiotherapy. It interferes with swallowing and taste, as well as denture retention and tolerance
◆ Increased duration of the oral preparatory phase of swallowing
◆ Increased dental caries, leading to tooth decay and potentially pain
◆ Burning mouth syndrome (stomatopyrosis) and burning tongue syndrome (glossopyrosis)
◆ Inflammation of the parotid salivary glands (suppurative parotitis)

Causes of reduced saliva

Reduced saliva is not age-related, yet up to 75 per cent of older people are affected (see below). Causes may include the following:

◆ Side effects of drugs (such as anticholinergics, antidepressants, Parkinsonian medication, motion sickness medication, continence medication, morphine). There tends to be an increase in the number of medications used with increasing age. It is helpful to liaise with the pharmacy team.
◆ Radiotherapy to head and neck, which also may cause inflammation of tissues. Irradiation of the salivary glands (sometimes used in the management of drooling) may have a permanent, irreversible effect, even up to three years later. This in turn may cause problems in oral care.

◆ Dehydration.

◆ Mouth breathing, continuous oxygen, or suction.

Suggested management techniques

◆ Chewing sugar-free sweets to create saliva flow.

◆ Rigorous oral care.

◆ Avoid or reduce caffeine, tobacco and alcohol (including any mouth rinse with a high alcohol content) as they are dehydrating. Acidic and highly seasoned foods may contribute to the problem.

◆ Artificial salivas. These physically resemble saliva but may lack its protective properties, although some contain fluoride. They are best applied to the reservoir under the tongue, not on the dorsum, as the client can then move the liquid around their own mouth. Currently available in the United Kingdom:

   – Only Luborant is licensed for any condition giving rise to dry mouth

   – Others commonly prescribed (for example, Glandosane, Saliva Orthana and MouthKote) are approved only for a dry mouth resulting from radiotherapy or connective tissue disease.

◆ Local measures: ice cubes, frozen tonic water, frozen fruit juice, pineapple chunks (contain a proteolytic enzyme, ananase, which also cleans the mouth; unsweetened tinned pineapple is preferable, which, if necessary, can be presented in gauze). If pain is a significant problem, a surface anaesthetic can be used with care.

Coping with drooling

Causes

Excess saliva often reflects reduction in the frequency of the automatic swallow, reduced oral sensation, and/or reduced tongue movement. The cause is rarely hypersalivation unless it is a side effect of protracted use of tranquillising or anticonvulsant medication.

Assessment

A drooling severity rating scale is included in Appendix IV. For various observation checklists, see Johnson and Scott (1993).

Management

Behaviour modification is the first line of approach in reducing drooling (Marks et al 2001b). Its primary goal is to increase the client's awareness of the saliva pooling in the mouth and/or drooling, in order that they consciously swallow more frequently. This may be achieved by asking the client to monitor their frequency of swallowing using a record chart for a fixed time period, say for five minutes, three times a day (see Appendix IV for an example). Clients who demonstrate some level of awareness often dab or wipe their lips to deal with dampness in the corners of their mouth or drooling. This dabbing or wiping may only stem the tide of saliva and may cause trauma to the skin. However, the dabbing or wiping can be used as a prompt for the client to elicit a swallow.

An alternative approach is to use a swallow reminder brooch (see Appendix II on suppliers). This small, portable device emits a beep at regular intervals (for example, every 27 seconds), reminding the client to swallow consciously (see Appendix IV for details of a programme). It may be useful to suggest that it is worn for 30 minutes each day for one month in order to obtain some carry-over into everyday situations.

If the individual experiences difficulty initiating a dry swallow, Logemann suggests a suck–swallow; that is, closing the lips, pumping the jaw and tongue to draw the saliva backwards, stimulating the swallow.

When pooling in the mouth or drooling is severe, particularly before eating or drinking, it may be helpful to encourage the client to perform a dry swallow before oral intake of food and/or drink commences. Oromotor exercises and stimulation of a delayed or absent swallow may be necessary to assist with this (see below).

For those who require a reduction in the quantity of saliva produced to decrease the risk of aspiration, the first management technique frequently employed is drug therapy. Medication that is given specifically to dry saliva includes the following:

◆ Scopolamine (Scopamine/Hyoscine) patches placed over the parotid gland. Alternatively, dilute drops can be applied under the tongue. The possibility of major central nervous system side-effects (such as sedation, confusion, restlessness, dizziness) occurring may limit its use, particularly where clients may have pre-existing cognitive change or confusion.

◆ Atropine, while less potent in blocking salivary secretions, has the benefit of less central nervous system suppression. It also appears to reduce the increased salivation that occurs in response to oesophageal reflux. The dose may be increased gradually to find the optimum.

◆ Bellafoline, like atropine, causes fewer side effects related to central nervous system suppression. Tolerance may develop in the longer term, resulting in a need to increase the dose, with a potential parallel increase in side-effects.

◆ Some find lemon and glycerine swabs beneficial. It is important to ensure that the mucosa does not become too dry. In addition, these swabs reduce the pH in the mouth to between 2 and 4 (acidic), which may decalcify teeth.

Permanent measures to reduce saliva production and drooling include surgery, such as salivary gland excision or rerouting the salivary ducts, and parotid radiotherapy. These techniques are best used when the strategies above were not beneficial, and the dysphagia is not resolving or is chronic. They may result in too dry mouth and complications of dental caries.

Dentures

There are two types of dentures. Complete (full) dentures replace the entire maxillary and/or mandibular dentition and its associated tissues. Modern ones are made of plastic (with a light pink colour covering the gums); a small number of upper dentures have a metal palate to strengthen the denture base. It is not uncommon for some older people to have had their dentures for 30 to 40 years. These often have a darker red material that covers the gums. A partial denture provides for a dental arch in which one or more remaining teeth may be accommodated.

Problems with dentures

Dentures are only one sixth as effective in chewing as natural teeth. New dentures may lead to a bitter and sour taste initially. This is normal, and usually resolves itself after one to two months, if the dentures are worn regularly. Altered sensation particularly occurs with an upper plate. They may cause reduced salivary flow initially. If the mouth is dry, it may help to use a fluoride mouthwash. New dentures need a five or six day bedding-in period, so start with soft food, then move to textures that require more chewing, and by day six to those that require biting. It is important that dentures are worn throughout this time, if possible.

Cleaning

Dentures may be cleaned using a toothbrush, twice a day, with cold water: too hot and they will warp. All denture-bearing areas (gums) need to be brushed also. A liquid unperfumed domestic soap may be used to clean all the surfaces of the denture. In addition, dentures may be soaked overnight in hypochlorite cleaning solution. Soaking alone (that is without brushing) is insufficient. For metal-based dentures, an alkaline peroxide solution is employed. Calculus (tartar) needs to be removed by a dentist or oral hygienist. When not in use, dentures are stored in cold water; otherwise the plastic will dry out and become distorted.

Maintenance

Regular dental examination is recommended: six-monthly for partial wearers, twelve-monthly for full wearers. The use of dental fixatives should only be a temporary measure and the cause of poor fitting remediated.

Removal

Dentures are removed at night to allow the mouth to recover from the denture-bearing load and to avoid a sore mouth, usually caused by a candidal infection of the soft tissues in contact with the denture, as a result of plaque and poor dental hygiene. If retained at night they must be scrupulously clean.

ORAL PREPARATORY AND ORAL STAGE REMEDIATION

This section will focus largely on indirect treatment (that is, oral control exercises), although direct management techniques (that is, giving food or drink with specific instructions) are also included.

The remediation of the oral preparatory and oral stages (as well as the pharyngeal stage) can be placed in a hierarchy as follows:

◆ Facilitation techniques – for absent or minimal movements

◆ Resistance – to increase the strength of movement

◆ Range of movement exercises – once reliable movement is achieved

◆ Strategies

Each level of this hierarchy may not be achievable for all aspects of the oral preparatory and oral stages. For example, the only area that is remediable if there is no movement is the lower facial musculature. For all other areas, some movement must emerge as a foundation for resistance or range of movement exercises to build upon.

Table 6.2 Oral Preparatory and Oral Stage Remediation		
ANATOMICAL AREA	*PROBLEM*	*REMEDIATION (see also Chapter 4)*
Jaw	Poor closure	Facilitated jaw support (see Figure 6.2)
	Chewing	Chew bags
Lips	Lower facial weakness	Orofacial facilitation (see text)
	Reduced lip strength	Resistance exercises: holding spatulas, puffing out cheeks
	Poor lip closure	Teeth to lip closure
Tongue	Protrusion	Bitter taste, pushing the tongue tip in gently, tapping tip, licking jam off lips
	Lateral movement	Catheter or liquorice lace, chew bag
	Tongue tip elevation	Polo on dental floss, licking chocolate from alveolar ridge
	Anterior–posterior movement	Sucking, gauze dipped in juice
	Tongue thrust	Guide tongue back, sucking
	Tongue pumping	Aim is to increase awareness and reduce in conjunction with improving the quality of anterior–posterior movement
	Residue	Increase awareness using tactile, visual and verbal prompts
	Control	Cohesive bolus

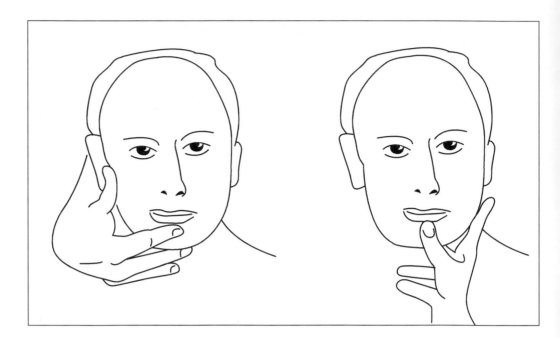

Figure 6.2
Two techniques for facilitated jaw closure

Orofacial facilitation (based on Kennedy 1989, unpublished)

◆ The aim is to combine a stimulation technique (icing), with a manipulation technique (pressure) to facilitate muscle movement. For maximum effect the programme is completed a minimum of three times a day.

◆ A piece of ice, the size of a lozenge, is wrapped in double thickness moist cotton gauze. It may be necessary to run the ice under a warm tap to achieve the correct size and ensure that it is smooth (see also Chapter 11 regarding health and safety issues).

◆ The muscle selected (see Figure 6.3) is stimulated by flicking with the ice, using five quick strokes. It is essential to flick in the direction the muscle moves. Always start at the top of the face and work down, since the effect radiates downwards.

◆ Using a pad of dry gauze, dab the area as soon as it has been iced. This is necessary to avoid ice burns. Use only one firm dab or the effect will be lost.

◆ Immediately guide the muscle into the desired movement using the fingertips, mirroring the movement on the unaffected side. Hold the position for three seconds.

◆ Repeat these steps twice more, and then move on to the next muscle group.

◆ Stop if the muscles start to tighten up.

◆ Remember: a facial weakness will appear asymmetrical if the unaffected side is overworking. Before commencing the programme, and at regular intervals

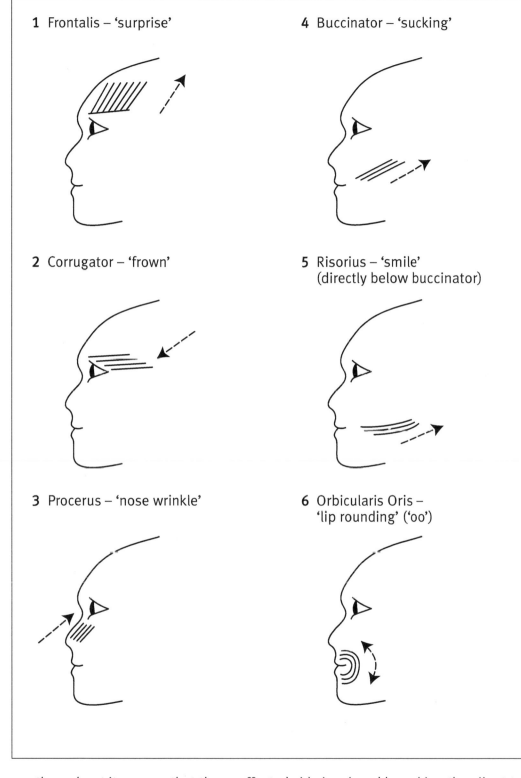

1 Frontalis – 'surprise'

4 Buccinator – 'sucking'

2 Corrugator – 'frown'

5 Risorius – 'smile'
(directly below buccinator)

3 Procerus – 'nose wrinkle'

6 Orbicularis Oris –
'lip rounding' ('oo')

Figure 6.3
Orofacial facilitation

throughout it, ensure that the unaffected side is relaxed by asking the client to spend time looking at themselves in a mirror, relaxing the unaffected side as much as possible.

Reduced or altered sensation is not remediable.

INTRODUCTION

A number of management techniques may be applied to more than one area of breakdown. In addition, it should be stressed that there is a significant overlap of assessment and management – what may be termed therapeutic assessment or continuing evaluative therapy.

COUGH

Chapter 3 (Subjective Assessment of Swallowing) provided information regarding the elicitation of a voluntary and/or reflexive cough. Since a reflexive cough relies on adequate sensation (which is not remediable) this is not an area to which therapy strategies can be applied. However, removing an agent such as a tracheostomy tube, which results in loss of sensation, may increase sensation.

Production of a voluntary cough is normally the focus of intervention when it is required to clear pooling of secretions or the bolus in the pyriform fossae, or on the vocal folds (see causes below) to reduce the risk of their being aspirated.

◆ If a voluntary cough is achievable and present, the client may benefit from feedback regarding its strength and efficiency, so that they can recognise when it is strong enough.

◆ The respiratory physiotherapist can teach a cooperative and cognitively aware client to produce a voluntary cough based on a technique known as huffing, or the huff and rattle.

◆ Deep breathing, vocal fold adduction exercises and phonosurgery (see below) may strengthen a volitional cough.

ABSENT OR DELAYED SWALLOW

Some of the techniques described below can assist both the stimulation of an absent swallow and the speed of triggering the swallow. A number only assist the latter. The majority of techniques are used in combination to maximise their effect.

Thermal stimulation (for both absent and delayed swallows)

This icing technique can be extremely effective. While the process is not fully understood, it is believed to prime the central nervous system ready for swallowing. It does not produce a 'knee jerk' reaction.

For an absent or significantly delayed swallow, we suggest that thermal stimulation be used intensively (that is, about five times a day) for a short period (two weeks). If there is no effect, it may be beneficial to discontinue, and then reinstate it for a further week, at which point, if there is no change, the programme is unlikely to work. Once the swallow is established, it may be used as a maintenance technique (to reduce delay) before and during meals. However it is used, clients or carers who act as proxy therapists require sufficient training to ensure that it is carried out effectively (see Chapter 13).

The programme can be used initially to elicit a dry swallow, moving on to the introduction of small quantities of oral intake, such as ice-cream and fluids. The overall aim is to develop the swallow to such an extent that the thermal stimulation is no longer required.

Equipment

You will need an '00'-sized laryngeal mirror, a damp wooden spatula, a pen torch, a cup containing ice (and a small quantity of water).

Procedure

1   Depress the tongue with the damp spatula (Figure 7.1), laying the pen torch along it so that the faucal arches are clearly visible.
2   Chill the mirror in the ice.
3   With the cold mirror, administer four to five light strokes at the base of one side of the anterior faucal arch. If the client gags, you are too far back (or the client has not been desensitised sufficiently – see Chapter 7, 'Oral Stage Management').
4   Re-chill the mirror, and then repeat on the other side.

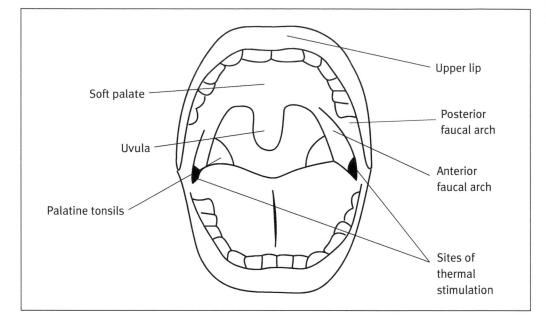

Figure 7.1
*Thermal
stimulation to
the anterior
faucal arch*

5 Ask the client to close their mouth and swallow (this may need to be demonstrated). Feel for or observe the swallow.

Frequency

Each session is likely to last five to ten minutes, with a minimum of five sessions a day. It may be possible to ask the carers to perform the programme as part of their regular observations, such as measuring blood pressure or temperature. Monitoring progress is essential. An example of a progress monitoring form is provided in Appendix IV.

Increase sensation (designed to reduce any delay in triggering the swallow)

The most commonly used technique to increase the stimulation of the swallow reflex is providing a chilled bolus. More recently it has been suggested that using fizzy drinks may provide a similar effect (Nixon, 1997). Alternatively, a sour bolus may be stimulating for demented and less alert clients. In our experience, sherry can have the same effect. Increasing the bolus size may facilitate triggering of the swallow. Conversely, reducing the speed and size of food presentation prevents severe collection of food in the pharynx and aspiration for some clients.

Increasing the cohesion of the bolus (to buy time for clients with a delayed swallow)

Thin liquids lose cohesion after a second; therefore, if a delay exists, provision of either naturally thicker or artificially thickened drinks is indicated. The level of thickening required is client-specific, dictated by the length of delay and the effectiveness of other strategies, such as chilling.

Using flexed head posture (to buy time for clients with a delayed swallow)

A flexed head position (Figure 7.2) increases control of the bolus in the pharynx since it

◆ Provides a wider vallecular space to hold the bolus

◆ Narrows the airway entrance, by bringing the tongue base closer to the posterior pharyngeal wall and pushing the epiglottis posteriorly, and

◆ Increases the length of cricopharyngeal opening

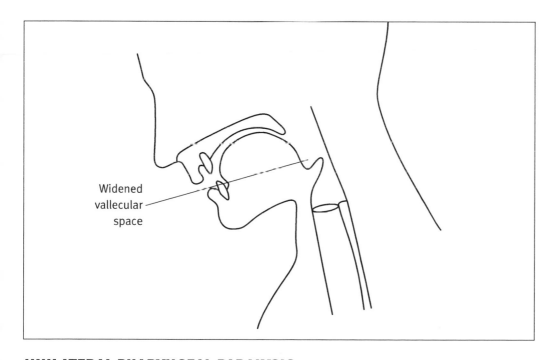

Figure 7.2
Head flexion to enhance the vallecular space

UNILATERAL PHARYNGEAL PARALYSIS

The pharynx may spontaneously compensate for this since 'Unilateral pharyngeal wall paresis causes the paralysed side to move towards the healthy side, Vernet's "mouvement de rideau"' (Hughes & Wiles, 1998). If the problem persists, two management options are available: (a) head turning towards the affected side, in order to close it off, or (b) head tilting to the unaffected side to take advantage of gravity carrying the bolus down the stronger side. The effectiveness of utilising these manoeuvres can be evaluated using videofluoroscopy or FEESS.

REDUCED VOCAL FOLD MOVEMENT

Reduced vocal fold movement (unilateral or bilateral) is diagnosed by listening to the client's voice quality and cough, and observations from videofluoroscopy or FEESS, or ENT assessment. Knowing the position of a paralysed vocal fold is helpful for selecting the appropriate strategy.

If both vocal folds are fixed in the midline, it will be necessary to insert a tracheostomy tube to permit breathing. (See Chapter 8 for details of the effects of tracheostomies on swallowing.)

Strategies to increase the safety of the swallow in the event of reduced vocal fold closure are detailed below.

Bolus consistency

Thickened liquids, purée and thick foods are helpful to prevent the bolus entering the airway before or during the swallow (Logemann, 1998).

Head flexion

This is an advisable strategy to implement for any client with reduced vocal fold adduction or closure. It increases protection of the airway by placing the epiglottis in a more overhanging position.

Head turn

Turning the head to the damaged side puts pressure on the damaged vocal fold, moving it slightly towards the midline to improve adduction. See also management of unilateral pharyngeal paralysis, above.

Supraglottic swallow

A supraglottic swallow puts vocal fold closure under cortical or voluntary control. Its purpose is to close the airway at the level of the vocal folds before and during the swallow, and to clear any residue from the pharynx after the swallow.

Instructions to the client are as follows:

1 Take a breath in.
2 Hold it.
3 Keep holding it while you swallow.
4 Cough before you take a breath.

It is essential to ensure that the client is actually holding their breath at the level of the larynx rather than simply arresting chest movement. This can be combined with head turning to the damaged side and/or a chin down posture. For a more detailed hierarchy to facilitate the use of the supraglottic swallow using food and drink, see Appendix IV.

Super supraglottic swallow

This development of the supraglottic swallow aims to close the entrance to the airway voluntarily by tilting the arytenoid cartilages anteriorally to increase tongue base movement. It is useful primarily for clients with penetration and/or aspiration after the swallow. It is not advised for clients with high blood pressure, as bearing down may aggravate their hypertension.

Instructions to the client are:

1 Take a breath in and hold it very tightly.
2 Bear down while you swallow.
3 Cough immediately after you swallow (before you take a breath).

Vocal fold adduction exercises

Examples:

- Say a prolonged 'ahhh'.
- Repeat 'ah' 10 times, making the voice as loud and smooth as possible.
- Take a deep breath, hold it tight, and say 'ah' for several seconds.
- Take a deep breath, hold it tight, and then cough loudly.
- Cough into 'ah'.

Phonosurgery for unilateral paralysis

Surgically adding additional mass to the damaged vocal fold facilitates closure by improving contact with the other, mobile fold. Logemann (1998) suggests that surgery not be performed until swallowing therapy has been trialled for a minimum of six months. This is because scar tissue can be more detrimental to the swallow. Types of surgery include the following:

- Thyroplasty or medialisation which can be achieved under local anaesthetic, to produce superior, yet reversible results should the problem resolve itself.
- Collagen injections, which may be suitable if only small gaps result from a vocal fold paralysis.
- Teflon injections, available for larger gaps; however the teflon may migrate, necessitating further surgery.
- Liposuction injection of abdominal fat, which has been reported to reduce aspiration by 100 per cent. The effects on voice quality may not be perfect.

REDUCED PHARYNGEAL PERISTALSIS

Clients who present with reduced pharyngeal peristalsis will experience increased problems as the consistency of the bolus becomes drier and more solid. The following strategies may be of value:

- More moist foods, for example using gravy, custard, cream.
- Dry, clearing swallows between mouthfuls.
- Alternating solids with fluids, but only if the swallow is otherwise competent, so that the client can cope with mixed consistencies.

REDUCED BASE OF TONGUE MOVEMENT

An effortful swallow can be used to improve tongue base movement and reduce residue in the valleculae post swallow. The client is instructed to swallow normally, but squeeze hard with the muscles of the tongue and throat. This excess effort should be visible in the neck, and may be combined with a chin-flexed posture (see above), which pushes the tongue base posteriorly into the pharynx. Alternatively, the blade of the tongue can be held between the front teeth and the client asked to swallow holding this position. The client will feel extra effort being exerted by the tongue base and posterior pharyngeal wall.

REDUCED LARYNGEAL ELEVATION

Reduced laryngeal elevation is most commonly associated with a brainstem CVA, or following head and neck surgery. The techniques suggested to encourage increased laryngeal elevation include the following:

◆ Falsetto. Ask the client to slide up a musical scale as high as possible and then hold it for several seconds. The client can monitor this elevation by feeling it with their hand.

◆ The Mendelsohn manoeuvre. The purpose of this technique is to accentuate and prolong laryngeal elevation, which results in an increase of the extent and duration of cricopharyngeal opening. The client is asked to swallow with their hand held to their larynx and feel its elevation. Next, they are asked to swallow again, but this time to hold the larynx up for a few seconds and not allow it to lower. Alternatively, they can be asked to 'hold the squeeze'. This prolongs the time that the larynx is most elevated, the tongue is most retracted in contact with the posterior pharyngeal wall, and the airway is closed (Logemann, 1998).

◆ Surface electromyography (EMG) which records muscle activity, using electrodes applied to the skin (see Chapter 4). This activity may then be converted into an auditory and visual display to provide targets and performance feedback for the client.

CRICOPHARYNGEAL DYSFUNCTION

Failure of the cricopharyngeus to open on swallowing is extremely rare. The problem is generally caused by incomplete laryngeal elevation, such that there is insufficient biomechanical pull to open the sphincter. The most common ways to increase cricopharyngeal opening are dilation or myotomy. A myotomy involves an external incision through the side of the neck into the cricopharyngeal muscle, slitting the fibres from top to bottom to open the sphincter permanently (Logemann, 1998). Logemann advises that this should not be performed early in the recovery of a client where the onset was acute, as most of these people will make a successful recovery. Management of this disorder is handed over to the ENT or gastroenterology team. Alternatively, Crary *et al* (1995) suggest that, as with many spasm disorders, there is potential in the use of transcutaneous injection of botulinum toxin. However, inaccurate injection can cause paralysis of other muscles in the area, potentially exacerbating the dysphagia (Logemann, 1998).

Chapter 8: Tracheostomies and Ventilators

INTRODUCTION

The purpose of this chapter is to serve as an introduction to the types of tracheostomy tubes and their effect on the respiratory and swallowing mechanisms, and to provide an overview of assessment and management for clients with a tracheostomy and those requiring mechanical ventilation. We strongly recommend that clinicians new to this particular area observe and work jointly with a more experienced clinician and, where they are available, physiotherapists, tracheostomy nurse specialists and ENT and intensive care colleagues, to develop further knowledge and skills. However experienced the clinician is, a multidisciplinary approach to assessment and management of swallowing with these clients is imperative. We suggest the following further reading:

◆ 'Managing tracheostomy and dysphagia' (Haynes & Hibberd, Autumn 1998);
◆ *Communication and Swallowing Management of Tracheostomized and Ventilator-Dependent Adults* (Dikeman & Kazandjian, 1995).

GENERAL ISSUES RELATED TO THE CARE OF CLIENTS WITH TRACHEOSTOMIES

These clients are at potential risk of complications that can be life threatening, which must not be ignored, whether in the ward or home environment. A blocked tracheostomy tube has serious consequences. Any concerns should be discussed, and advice sought from experienced clinicians. With the appropriate level of care these complications can be prevented.

MAINTENANCE OF THE AIRWAY

Clients need to maintain a patent airway and a clear chest in order to breathe efficiently. If the airway becomes too narrow, for example owing to burns or surgical oedema, and/or the client is unable to cough effectively, for example because of a unilateral vocal fold palsy, secretions may accumulate in the chest and an artificial airway may need to be inserted in order to perform suction. An airway can be provided with an oral (Figure 8.1) or nasal endotracheal tube, or with a tracheostomy tube (Figure 8.2). Ventilators provide mechanical ventilation.

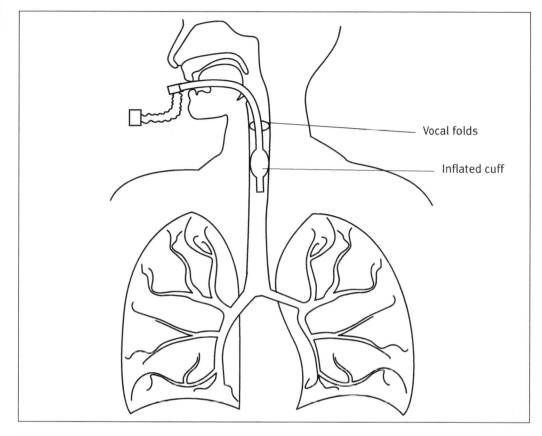

Figure 8.1
Position of an endotracheal tube for oral intubation

Vocal folds

Inflated cuff

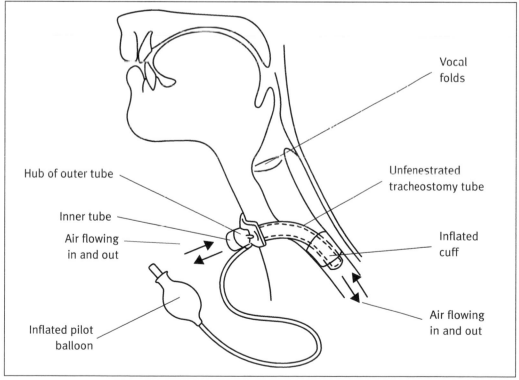

Vocal folds

Hub of outer tube

Inner tube

Air flowing in and out

Unfenestrated tracheostomy tube

Inflated cuff

Inflated pilot balloon

Air flowing in and out

Figure 8.2
Components of an unfenestrated tracheostomy tube

Although endotracheal intubation is performed as an emergency (for example following a respiratory arrest), most admissions to the intensive care unit are electively ventilated (for example, clients who undergo cardiac or head and neck surgery are ventilated during surgery and afterwards on intensive care wards for a period of time). The tube may be left in place for hours, days or weeks, depending on the nature and severity of the client's medical or surgical condition. Insertion of the tube and its presence for any length of time can result in laryngeal and tracheal trauma. The movement of the tube and cuff against the laryngeal and tracheal mucosa causes tissue irritation and potential abrasion. Complications include the following:

◆ Laryngeal and/or supraglottic oedema

◆ Glottic incompetence (see below)

◆ Formation of laryngeal nodules, polyps, granulomas or haematomas

◆ Unilateral laryngeal or adductor paresis or paralysis

◆ Laryngeal stenosis (narrowing of the laryngeal inlet, this is rare, but serious)

◆ Trauma caused by the bottom end of the tube rubbing against the posterior tracheal wall, leading to breakdown in the tissue which may result in a tracheosophageal fistula. This is a rare, but serious, event

Swallowing assessment or intervention is not indicated until the oral or nasal endotracheal intubation is removed. The client may be receiving nasogastric feeding (see Chapter 10). When the endotracheal tube is removed, the client may have a degree of hoarseness and/or stridor, which generally resolves spontaneously. If these do not resolve, referral to ENT colleagues is indicated. Dikeman and Kazandjian (1995) suggest that endotracheal tubes affect the tongue base, and that a transient dysphagia may result post removal.

GLOTTIC INCOMPETENCE

The normal laryngeal protective responses can be affected by the presence of long-term endotracheal intubation or a tracheostomy tube. Examples of these protective responses are laryngeal closure and the ability to clear aspirated material from the larynx or trachea. These responses are disrupted because the sensory receptors under the vocal folds are not stimulated by air flowing over the larynx, which may result in aspiration of saliva and oral intake (Dikeman & Kazandjian, 1995). Glottic incompetence may also apply to actual structural damage to the vocal folds. This may be resolved by ensuring that air is redirected through the larynx (for example by using a fenestrated tracheostomy tube with a speaking valve – see below), allowing time for spontaneous recovery and the use of appropriate therapeutic exercises (see Chapter 7). Referral to ENT colleagues is particularly necessary when glottic incompetence is suspected, so as to confirm the diagnosis (using fibre-optic nasendoscopy and FEESS if appropriate – see Chapter 4) and to promote appropriate management, for example voice rest.

INDICATIONS FOR A TRACHEOSTOMY

A percutaneous tracheostomy is normally a temporary and occasionally a permanent opening into the anterior wall of the trachea, below the vocal folds to prevent damaging the larynx. It may be inserted for various medical or surgical reasons. Such reasons will influence the type of tube required and the care the client will need. Common reasons for tracheostomy insertion include the following:

◆ Respiratory failure.

◆ Raised intracranial pressure, resulting in reduced ability to control oxygenation and carbon dioxide status.

◆ Provision of an alternative airway where there is a risk of acute or chronic airway obstruction at or above the level of the vocal folds, for example in an unconscious client who has undergone neurosurgery and requires prolonged ventilation via an endotracheal tube (this can result in laryngeal and pharyngeal oedema), or a client with a head injury and multiple facial fractures which require surgery that can result in post-operative oedema of the surrounding tissues.

◆ The need to bypass an actual upper airway obstruction, such as bilateral abductor vocal fold palsy or subglottic stenosis resulting from prolonged endotracheal ventilation.

◆ Long-term airway or ventilatory requirements, such as in Guillain-Barré disease, motor neurone disease, spinal cord injuries and weaning long-term clients from the ventilator.

◆ Protection against aspiration of oral secretions or diet in clients who have an ineffective swallow, for example following brainstem stroke.

◆ Provision of respiratory care and pulmonary toilet or suction. Reilly and Carroll (1992) describe the latter as the removal of excess secretions from the respiratory tract by the insertion of a catheter into the tracheostomy or endotracheal tube and applying negative pressure by occluding the proximal port of the suction catheter. It is used when clients retain sputum in the lungs and are unable to cough effectively. The authors state that it is 'a potentially dangerous procedure for the trained person to perform and should never be carried out by untrained personnel or without adequate supervision in the case of training'.

Secretions that pool above the cuff (see below) have been identified as a cause of ventilator-associated pneumonia. In a similar vein, it is important to note that positioning a client supine (lying on the back) also has a higher incidence of ventilator-associated pneumonia (Goldstone, 2000).

The client's comfort is increased with a tracheostomy rather than an oral or nasal endotracheal tube. Other benefits of tracheostomy tube placement are increased opportunities for communication and oral intake. A tracheostomy tube usually remains in place until the airway obstruction, the potential for obstruction and the need for respiratory care (ventilation and/or suctioning) have subsided.

TYPES OF TRACHEOSTOMY TUBES

Tracheostomies are either disposable (made of plastic, being softer and more comfortable) or non-disposable (made of metal, very rigid and heavy but reusable if sterilised). The latter are generally not used for clients requiring mechanical ventilation, as they do not have cuffs. Disposable tracheostomy tubes may have a single or double cannula and can be

◆ Cuffed
◆ Cuffless
◆ Unfenestrated (see Figure 8.2)
◆ Fenestrated (see Figure 8.3)
◆ A cricothyroidotomy tube and minitracheostomy (these have a single cannula)

A cuffed tube is used when mechanical ventilation is required and when there is the potential to aspirate oral secretions. A fenestrated tube allows air to pass up through the vocal folds, permitting phonation, and facilitates swallowing assessment and management as the client's voice quality can be monitored.

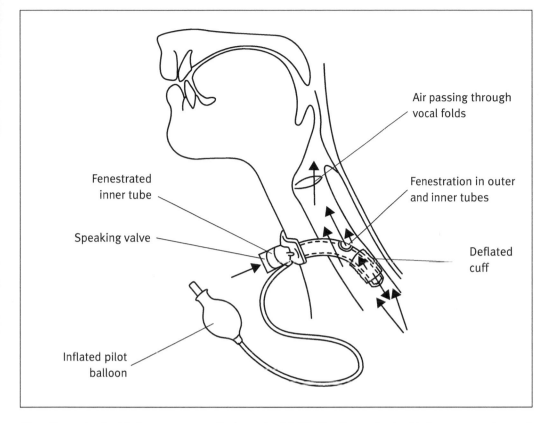

Air passing through vocal folds

Fenestrated inner tube

Speaking valve

Fenestration in outer and inner tubes

Deflated cuff

Inflated pilot balloon

Figure 8.3
A fenestrated cuffed tracheostomy tube with the cuff deflated and a speaking valve in situ, demonstrating air passing up through the vocal folds

Non-fenestrated tubes are usually inserted initially. Fenestrated tubes are not used with clients who are at high risk of aspiration because of the risk of secretions or oral intake passing through the fenestration into the trachea and potentially into the lower airway. Fenestrated tubes are inserted as part of the weaning or decannulation process – that is, the removal of the tracheostomy. It is usual for the fenestrated tracheostomy tube to be supplied with two inner cannulas. One of the inner cannulas is unfenestrated and is inserted into the outer tube when suction is required, as the suction catheter can become stuck in the fenestration and cause mechanical trauma to the trachea or vocal folds. The other inner cannula is fenestrated and is used for phonation. Having two inner cannulas permits one to be worn while the other is cleaned. This prevents the tube from becoming obstructed by sputum plugs.

A cricothyroidotomy tube is usually inserted in an emergency when the client's anatomy will not permit the creation of a tracheostomy stoma and an airway is required. It involves inserting a narrower lumen tube in the midline of the cricothyroid membrane. Its disadvantage is that injury to the trachea and larynx may occur, as the incision is made higher up than a tracheostomy. A minitracheostomy tube may be inserted into the stoma where a tracheostomy was as part of the weaning procedure (see later in this chapter).

The physician's knowledge of the client's general anatomy, weight and potential to aspirate, as well as the length of the tube, governs the size and type of the tube selected. The physician selects the appropriate sized tube that will (a) provide the client with as large an airway as possible for ventilation, (b) have a low risk of tracheal abrasion, and (c) allow sufficient airflow round the sides of the tube and the lumen of the trachea. When ventilation is no longer required, Dikeman and Kazandjian (1995) suggest that 'the tracheostomy tube should fill no more than two thirds to three quarters of the tracheal lumen'. The type and size of tube is normally found on the flange or on the pilot balloon. Information as to whether the tube is cuffed or cuffless, fenestrated or unfenestrated is found on the flange.

THE IMPACT OF A TRACHEOSTOMY ON SECRETION CONTROL AND OTHER FUNCTIONS

The normal warming, filtering and humidification of the inhaled air is disrupted owing to the presence of a tracheostomy tube and, as a result, the lower respiratory tract is more vulnerable to irritants (Dikeman & Kazandjian, 1995). The disruption of normal airflow through the upper respiratory tract during inhalation and exhalation results in reduced evaporation of oral secretions, which then accumulate in the mouth. This increased volume of secretions is more difficult to clear, as the cough reflex is less effective when a tracheostomy is present. This is because air is unable to reach the vocal folds, and so the air pressure needed to forcefully eject the accumulated mucus is reduced and will necessitate oral and tracheal suctioning.

As explained earlier, when air no longer flows over the larynx for extended periods the sensitivity of the larynx is reduced, resulting in an impaired glottic closure response. This may lead to chronic aspiration without eliciting a glottal closure response: that is, silent aspiration (Nash, 1988). In addition, this disrupted airflow affects the client's ability to smell and taste.

THE IMPACT OF A TRACHEOSTOMY ON SWALLOWING

The potential for dysphagia is increased when a client has a tracheostomy tube because of the effects of the sensory and respiratory impairments consequent of the presence of a tracheostomy tube. Clients with compromised respiratory systems are at greater risk from pulmonary infections and so the impact of aspiration is more severe. The tracheostomy tube can have (a) a mechanical and (b) a physiological impact on swallowing function.

Mechanical impact

There may be reduced laryngeal elevation: the larynx becomes anchored, and so full laryngeal elevation may be difficult to achieve. If the client is ventilated, the ventilator tubing may tether the larynx further. Logemann (1998) reports that the larynx in older clients (over the age of 80) rests lower in the neck and this further reduces elevation.

Problems associated with cuff inflation include the following:

1   Groher (1992) suggests that 'if a patient's medical condition is so precarious that a cuffed tracheostomy tube is warranted, perhaps oral feeding is premature'.

2   It may be common for some physicians to recommend that clients eat with the cuff inflated. This is due to the belief that the cuff reduces the risk of aspiration as any material aspirated below the level of the larynx will remain above the cuff and not enter the lower airway. However, this is not necessarily the case, as videofluoroscopy studies demonstrate that the bolus can slip down between the inflated cuff and the tracheal walls.

3   The inflated cuff can reduce laryngeal elevation by creating friction against the tracheal wall (Logemann, 1998). Logemann suggests that swallowing with an inflated cuff interferes with swallowing rehabilitation and recovery. However, for some clients (such as those in the end stages of motor neurone disease), eating with the cuff up may be recommended.

4   It prevents the production of an effective cough clearing the larynx. In addition, if the client is aspirating food or fluids, it is crucial to know immediately so that suction may be performed promptly. An inflated cuff delays this knowledge (see Figure 8.2), as the bolus may be slow to seep through the narrow gap between the cuff and the trachea wall.

5 An overinflated cuff can impinge on the oesophagus, disturbing peristalsis and leading to a partial blockage of the oesophagus, so that the food backs up to the pharynx and may be observed around the outer cannula at the stoma site (see Figure 8.4).

Physiological impact

◆ *Disruption of airway pressures.* Dikeman and Kazandjian (1995) describe how the base of tongue movement creates airway pressure that drives the bolus through the pharynx and into the oesophagus. After the cricopharyngeus relaxes, the pressures shift into the oesophagus. 'An open tracheostomy tube disrupts the maintenance of these pressures and will result in the accumulation of residue in the pharynx.'

◆ *Reduction of airflow through the glottis.* This has three effects. First, expiration cannot function in its usual way, that is to clear residue from the airway. Second, the gradual loss of laryngeal sensation blunts the reflexive cough, which becomes increasingly ineffective. Third, the glottic or laryngeal closure response during the swallow becomes delayed, resulting in the bolus entering between or below the vocal folds that move sluggishly.

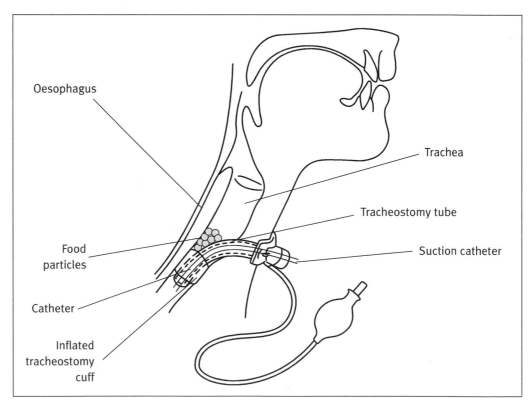

Figure 8.4
Aspirated food pooled above an inflated tracheostomy cuff

MANAGEMENT OF A TRACHEOSTOMY CUFF

'A decrease in cilia has been identified at the cuff inflation site. Cilia are necessary for the removal of mucus and aspirated contents from the airway. The reduction of cilia eliminates yet another level of protection from the tracheostomised and ventilator-dependent patient' (Dikeman & Kazandjian, 1995).

If the cuff is overinflated with air (injected via a syringe, into the pilot balloon), the tracheal walls around the cuff begin to soften and break down (see Figure 8.5). This results in the loss of the seal between the cuff and the tracheal wall. As the space around the cuff is larger, an air leak results. A vicious circle then develops in that, to obtain a seal, the health professional injects more air into the pilot balloon. 'Tracheomalacia' is the term given to the softening of the rings of cartilage of the trachea caused by repeated trauma. The trachea can then collapse inwards during the inspiratory phase of breathing. It is most important that clinicians be aware of these potential complications, as they may be involved in cuff deflation and reinflation as part of their assessment and management of the client's dysphagia.

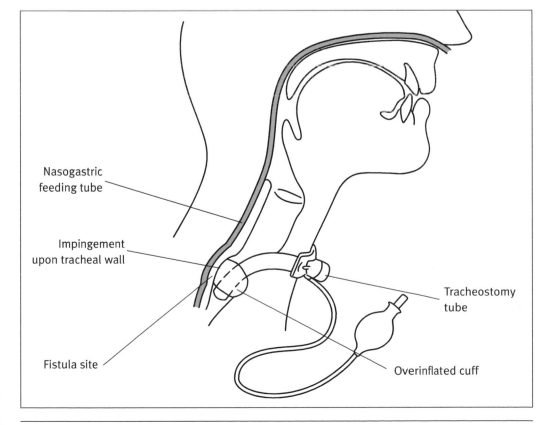

Nasogastric feeding tube

Impingement upon tracheal wall

Fistula site

Tracheostomy tube

Overinflated cuff

Figure 8.5
Complications of an over-inflated cuff

Overinflation of the cuff can be prevented by using a cuff manometer (available on intensive care units and in ENT departments), or by using one of two techniques: minimal occluding volume or minimal leak. The first involves slowly injecting air into the cuff while the client slowly exhales through the mouth and nose. Listening with a stethoscope on the lateral boarder of the thyroid cartilage, the clinician stops injecting air when no more air is heard on inhalation and exhalation, as a seal is assumed. Minimal leak uses the same technique, but has an additional stage. This involves the removal of a small volume of air from the pilot balloon, creating a minimal leak.

ASSESSMENT OF SWALLOWING WITH A CLIENT WITH A TRACHEOSTOMY TUBE

The assessment of swallowing for a client with a tracheostomy is essentially the same as any dysphagia assessment, in terms of gathering of information from the medical history, client and carers (see Chapters 3 and 4). The client's nurse and/or physiotherapist's participation in the assessment is essential. They provide important assessment information on the client. Additional benefits are that they will have the opportunity to observe the strategies used, which can then be reinforced later. The clinical dysphagia evaluation is modified in various ways, as outlined below.

Haynes and Hibberd (1998) developed a tracheostomy checklist in conjunction with a physiotherapist. It provides a standard procedure based on clinical evidence. Part 1 of the form relates to information gathering, including details of the client's respiratory status and the type of ventilation. 'If it is felt that it is unsafe to carry out a swallowing assessment, the reasons should be documented in the patient's medical notes' (Haynes & Hibberd, 1998). If it is safe to continue the assessment further, information regarding the type of tracheostomy tube, the frequency of suctioning and the client's ability to tolerate cuff deflation are documented in Part 2. However, before continuing with the assessment, the clinician will discuss with the medical team whether they agree that the cuff may be deflated for assessment purposes. If the cuff needs to remain inflated during the assessment, the clinician should note this in the case notes and the initial report. We suggest the following procedure for cuff deflation, which is performed with the assistance of a physiotherapist or nurse who is experienced in suctioning. (Again, the clinician may decide that, if the client has excessive secretions and cannot tolerate cuff deflation, it may be best to stop the assessment at this point and until these difficulties resolve.)

If there is concern that the client is aspirating their saliva, a blue dye test may be performed prior to assessment on food or fluids (see Appendix IV). Dikeman and Kazandjian (1995) suggest that three blue dye tests be performed as 'The results of this test should be interpreted conservatively and monitored carefully, as experience indicates it is not wholly reliable' (Haynes & Hibberd, 1998). The general bedside observations of clinical predictors of aspiration will also be utilised.

Procedure for assessing swallowing with a client with a cuffed, fenestrated tracheostomy tube

◆ Suction above and below the level of the tracheostomy cuff, that is, at the back of the mouth and down the tracheostomy tube.

◆ Allow the client to rest.

◆ Insert the syringe into the pilot balloon and deflate the cuff slowly.

◆ Note how much air was removed.

◆ The client may cough on any secretions that were pooled above the cuff and not fully suctioned the first time. If this coughing does not settle, reinflate the cuff and suction again. Then deflate the cuff, if appropriate.

◆ Insert the fenestrated inner cannula.

◆ Ask the client to breathe in and out through their mouth to encourage air to pass through the glottis.

◆ Using a gloved finger, gently occlude the stoma while the client exhales. Ensure that this does not adversely affect their breathing and cause distress. If this is successful, occlude the stoma for a few seconds.

◆ Encourage the client to phonate on 'ahhhhh', note the voice quality, for example, wet-hoarse.

◆ Note the ability to cough to command or the strength of a reflex cough.

- If phonation is possible, trial the wearing of a speaking valve (for example, Rusch or Passy-Muir valve) during the assessment to facilitate glottic closure during swallowing. If the client is aphonic and the clinician is unable to ascertain whether this is due to the tube size or vocal fold movement, an ENT opinion should be sought.

- Ask the client to perform a dry swallow with the speaking valve in place, or suggest they occlude the stoma with their finger. Observe for any delay or reduction in laryngeal elevation.

- Place a few drops of blue food colouring on the client's tongue or in 1ml of sterile water allowing it to mix with the client's saliva, which may then be swallowed if possible (this can be continued every four hours for 48 hours, see Appendix IV).

- Perform routine tracheostomy care. Any evidence of blue dye in the tracheostomy aspirate or around the stoma itself is evidence of aspiration. Nash (1988) reported that the average time until a positive test result was confirmed was seven hours.

- If there is no evidence of aspiration of the client's oral secretions, proceed with the swallowing assessment as with a non-tracheostomised client, but using blue dyed thin, thick and semi-solid consistencies as appropriate (see Chapter 4).

- Observe for compounding factors such as respiratory fatigue, increased respiratory effort and respiratory rate.

- Note the presence and timing of a cough, change in voice quality and the client's awareness of the sound of the voice. In addition, note their ability to clear any penetrated or aspirated material with a clearing cough and/or swallow, whether this is spontaneous or follows verbal prompts. These strategies will be utilised in their management.

- Continue to monitor for signs of fatigue and aspiration during the assessment.

- Perform suctioning as necessary.

- Reinflate the cuff with the same volume of air as was removed, or use the minimal occluding volume or minimal leak techniques outlined earlier.

- Recommendations regarding management may include consistencies, quantities, frequency, length of time that the cuff is deflated and use of a speaking valve or cap.

◆ Ask the multidisciplinary team to continue to monitor for signs of aspiration, and to record the results of suctioning on a tracking sheet (see Dikeman & Kazandjian, 1995).

Cervical auscultation, FEESS and videofluoroscopy may be used as adjuncts to the clinical evaluation of swallowing (see Chapter 4).

ASSESSMENT OF SWALLOWING WITH A CLIENT WHO IS DEPENDENT ON A MECHANICAL VENTILATOR USING A PASSY-MUIR SPEAKING VALVE (from the Passy-Muir valve instruction booklet, supplied by Kapitex)

The silastic membrane of the Passy-Muir valve (PMV) maintains a closed position all the time except during inspiration, redirecting the exhaled air around the tracheostomy tube, through the vocal folds, mouth and nose, allowing the client to speak, swallow, smell and taste. Currently, this is the only speaking valve for use with ventilators. This is because it has the feature of positive closure. To function properly, the cuff needs to be fully deflated.

The PMV is contraindicated in clients who have severe tracheal or laryngeal obstruction; who have excessive and unmanageable pulmonary secretions and are unable to tolerate cuff deflation; who are unconscious or have no communicative intent; who have a bilateral vocal fold palsy (where the folds are fixed in the midline); or who are known to aspirate severely.

In our experience, the client is more likely to tolerate cuff deflation if the pressure support is 15 or less and the positive end expiratory pressure (PEEP) is five or less. Pressure support is the addition of pre-set positive pressure breaths to the inspiratory phase of ventilation. Its purpose is to help reduce the effort of breathing. PEEP is the maintenance of airway pressures above atmospheric throughout the expiratory phase of the ventilator. It helps by improving oxygenation. (For further explanation, see Dikeman and Kazandjian, 1995). The client is more likely to tolerate cuff deflation if the pressure support is 15 or less, because the increased rate and flow with high pressures cause discomfort.

The benefits of using a Passy-Muir valve are as follows:

- *Improved swallowing.* Positive closure restores the client to a more normal closed system, which facilitates increased pharyngeal/laryngeal sensation and restores positive subglottic air pressure. Thus the safety and efficiency of the swallow may be improved and aspiration reduced. The clinician will use clinical judgement to ascertain whether this is the case for each individual client.
- *Olfaction.* An improved sense of smell and taste is achieved as the air is diverted into the nasal passages. This may stimulate appetite and increase calorie intake.
- *Speech.* Clients can produce clearer speech with more normal phrasing, better vocal quality and increased volume. This allows the monitoring of voice quality during swallowing assessment and management.
- *Secretion management.* The valve's positive closure 'no leak' design facilitates secretion management as it re-establishes a 'closed system' that enables the client to produce a stronger cough. It also facilitates evaporation of oral secretions through the redirection of air through the upper airway during exhalation.

To assess the client's swallowing ability, it is essential that the clinician first obtains the physician's consent to deflate the cuff. A joint assessment is often carried out with the assistance of the client's nurse and/or physiotherapist. They assist with positioning, suctioning, cuff deflation, and monitoring the client's responses during the procedure (that is, respiratory status, vital signs, oxygenation, cardiac rhythm and ventilator changes). The nurse and physiotherapist assess the client and the ventilator settings; place the Passy-Muir valve in line (see Figure 8.6); adjust the ventilator to compensate for leakage (for example, tidal volume, pressure support, fraction of inspired oxygen and rate – see Dikeman & Kazandjian, 1995); set the appropriate volume and pressure alarms, monitor the client's responses, and document the trial. The speech and language therapist's role is to provide reassurance during cuff deflation, as this can produce anxiety in the client; to assist the client with phonation; to provide teaching related to the PMV; to assess swallowing in conjunction with PMV use, and to document the trial.

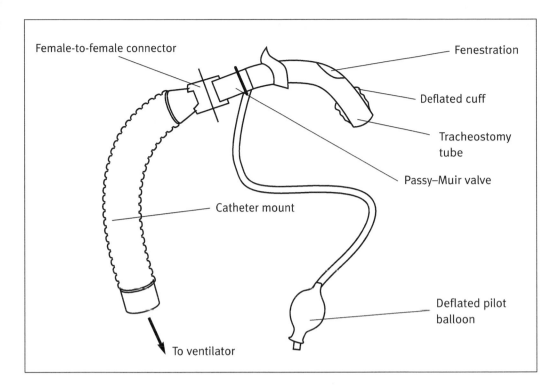

Female-to-female connector

Fenestration

Deflated cuff

Tracheostomy tube

Passy–Muir valve

Catheter mount

Deflated pilot balloon

To ventilator

Figure 8.6
Placement of a Passy-Muir valve with a ventilator-dependent client

The trial will last as long as the client tolerates the PMV, or as agreed by the assessing multidisciplinary team. Depending on the outcome of the trial, recommendations are made regarding PMV use and safety of oral intake. Despite changing of the ventilator settings, some clients do not tolerate the PMV. Bell (1996) outlines the following criteria for determining whether a trial is unsuccessful:

◆ Arterial blood oxygen saturation less than 90 per cent, or a decrease of more than 5 per cent from baseline reading (measured using a pulse oximeter or obtaining arterial blood and analysing the levels of oxygen and carbon dioxide dissolved in it).

◆ Respiratory rate increase of more than 10 breaths per minute from baseline.

◆ Significant change in blood pressure or heart rate (that is, plus or minus 10 per cent from baseline).

◆ Dyspnoea, anxiety or shortness of breath.

◆ Constant, uncontrollable coughing.

MANAGEMENT OF SWALLOWING FOR CLIENTS WITH TRACHEOSTOMIES

The management strategies outlined in Chapters 5, 6, 7 and 9 can be applied to these clients (for example, thickened fluids, head turn to the affected side, supraglottic swallow, Mendelsohn manoeuvre). In particular, rigorous oral hygiene is needed to prevent anaerobic bacteria in the mouth from moving past the cuff into the airway, resulting in 'microaspirations' (Dikeman & Kazandjian, 1995). Written guidelines are especially beneficial for teaching any specific mealtime strategies. Boolkin (1998) states that 'swallowing disorders following tracheostomy have been found to be extremely amenable to therapy, and thus the availability of a therapist during and after the intubation period may help shorten the course of such disorders'.

THE WEANING PROCESS FOR REMOVING THE TRACHEOSTOMY TUBE: DECANNULATION

The multidisciplinary team will discuss the client's readiness for removal of the tracheostomy tube. Principles to consider when planning weaning may include deflating the cuff for increasing lengths of time, until it is down continually. It may be appropriate to change the tube to (a) a smaller size to facilitate oral-nasal breathing in combination with breathing through the tracheostomy stoma, (b) an uncuffed tube, and/or (c) a fenestrated tube. A speaking valve, button or cap can be put in place for an increasing length of time, as tolerated, to facilitate mouth and nose breathing. It is helpful to ask the client and carers to note if and how frequently suctioning is required, or, whether difficulty in breathing occurred, necessitating the removal for comfort of the valve or cap. The time required for the tube to be occluded before removal ranges from two to 48 hours, day and night without requiring suction or the removal of the valve or cap. It is also helpful to consider the client's ability to prevent aspiration of secretions and the strength and effectiveness of the cough. ENT or appropriately trained staff generally remove the tracheostomy tube.

'Food isn't just about carbohydrates and calories. It is also about sociability, nurturing, stimulation of the sense through tastes and textures, creativity, sharing and pampering – in effect communication in its broadest sense.' (Onslow, 1999)

THE NUTRITIONAL TEAM

As stated in Chapter 5, helping the client meet their nutritional and hydration needs is a team responsibility. It is the most cost-effective management approach and results in fewer complications. Core members of the team include the client, their family and carers, nurses (both on a ward and district nurses in the community), the catering department, the dietitian, medical staff, pharmacy staff and the speech and language therapist. Some teams include a nutrition nurse specialist, to advise and educate on nursing aspects of nutritional support – enteral and parenteral (see below).

The dietitian is often recognised as the nutritional team leader. She is the most effective link to the diet kitchen to ensure the provision of appropriate modified food textures. Early input from the dietitian may prevent medical complications, such as pressure sores or dry mouth. Her involvement is essential if dysphagia exists, since poor nutritional and/or hydration status will have a marked impact on the efficiency of the swallow.

DAILY NUTRITIONAL REQUIREMENTS

Undernutrition reduces the client's capacity to deal with infection, increasing morbidity and lengthening the hospital admission. A basic guide to the daily nutritional targets for normal healthy adults is given below:

Milk	$\frac{1}{2}$–1 pint per day
Meat/fish/cheese/eggs/pulses	at least 2–3 portions of protein foods per day
Bread/breakfast cereals/pasta/rice/potatoes	at least 1 portion at each meal
Vegetables/salad/fruit/fruit juice	aim for 5 portions per day
Fluids	at least 8 cups per day

These figures will increase for older people and those who are medically unwell.

ASSESSING INTAKE AND NUTRITIONAL STATUS

A number of service areas in the United Kingdom have developed nutritional assessment tools for their specific client group, to screen for risk of malnutrition and identify which members of the team the client should be referred to. Such tools include assessment of physical condition, mental condition, history of unintentional weight loss, limitations on food/fluid intake, proportion of food consumed and increased nutritional needs (due, for example, to presence of infection, pressure sores, COPD, carcinoma, recent major surgery).

Nutritional tools may not be available for all client groups or service areas (such as adults with learning difficulties), but alternatives are available. The information gathered may be forwarded to the dietitian who can then determine whether further action is indicated. Owing to the limited provision of a dietetics service to clients in the community within the United Kingdom, the speech and language therapist may gather and share this information with the dietitian, as part of their dysphagia assessment:

◆ *Weight and height*, including information about perceived weight loss, for example asking whether the client's clothes have become looser or now require a belt to keep them up.

◆ *A 24-hour dietary history*. This can take the form of a written diary, such as food or fluid charts (useful in combination with a record of any swallowing difficulties encountered), or can be elicited by asking non-leading questions to gather this information (for example, 'What was the first thing you ate/drank this morning?').

◆ *Anthropometric measures*. These assess body mass, normally utilising mid-arm or calf circumferences to estimate a client's body weight. Following basic training, speech and language therapists can carry out these measures in the community, where weighing scales are not normally readily available.

NUTRITION AND HYDRATION SUPPORT

Clients with a depressed appetite, increased nutrient requirements that cannot be met by oral food/fluid alone, an inability to take food/fluid orally, and/or failure of the gastrointestinal tract, may require nutrition support to ensure that they meet their daily requirements. A number of methods are available, depending on the cause and severity of the underlying problem:

◆ Fortifying foods and drinks
◆ Supplements
◆ Alternative feeding routes
◆ Sluids
◆ Transitional feeding
◆ Strategies
◆ Medication

Fortifying foods and drinks

Simple strategies increase the energy and/or protein content of a food or drink while maintaining the normal portion size:

	Increases Energy	Increases Protein
Adding skimmed milk powder to milk which can then be used as normal	✓	✓
Cream/evaporated milk/yogurt	✓	
Butter/margarine	✓	
Cheese	✓	✓
Mayonnaise	✓	
Sugar/glucose	✓	
Jam/honey/lemon curd/marmalade	✓	

Hospital catering departments often offer high-protein options, which are usually marked on the menu ordering cards.

Supplements

A range of dietary supplements are available, normally on prescription. They may or may not be nutritionally complete, and are produced as powders (protein or glucose-based powders), liquids (carbohydrate or fat), fortified drinks (sip feeds), fortified soups (savoury versions of sip feeds) and puddings. They are used to supplement normal food and/or fluid intake rather than as a replacement. It is important for the clinician to have sampled the supplements used within their service, to ensure that they are aware of the reasons for potential client non-compliance in their use. Sip feeds are more palatable if chilled, and some can be incorporated into sorbets and ice creams. Adding a small amount of liqueur or spirits can improve the flavour. The consistency of many sip feeds may make them suitable for clients with dysphagia, without further thickening being required.

The cost of modifying menus or providing supplements has been estimated to be one-third that of enteral feeding per week, and one-fourteenth of the cost of parenteral feeding (see below) (*Drug and Therapeutics Bulletin*, 1996).

Alternative feeding routes

Feeding tubes may benefit clients when they provide time to treat underlying medical problems or to clarify prognosis, or when prolongation of life is feasible and desirable. There are two forms of tube feeding – enteral and parenteral – both of which deliver nutritionally complete liquid feeds.

Enteral tube feeding is suitable for clients with a normally functioning gastrointestinal tract, but who either are unable to take food and fluids orally or lack the motivation or ability to obtain enough energy and nutrients orally to meet their nutritional requirements. There are four enteral feeding routes:

1   *Fine bore nasogastric, or NG, tubes.* Normally for short-term use, an NG tube
    is inserted through the nose, through the pharynx and oesophagus into the
    stomach. Trained nurses and doctors can insert them, although they do
    require the client to swallow, which permits the opening of the
    cricopharyngeus, allowing the tube to enter the oesophagus.
2   *Fine bore nasoduodenal/jejunal tubes* are used in an identical way to NG
    tubes, but for patients with abnormal gastric function, or if there is a greater
    risk of aspiration of the refluxed feed. They are less commonly used.
3   *Percutaneous endoscopic gastrostomy feeding tubes, or PEGs,* are
    recommended for long-term feeding where part or full oral feeding is unlikely

to resume within two to three weeks. They are inserted into the abdomen endoscopically in a hospital theatre, necessitating client sedation. They require replacement every two years on average.

4 *Percutaneous jejunal feeding tubes (PEJs)* are inserted if there is concern about aspiration of refluxed feed or abnormal gastric function.

Parenteral nutrition (alternatively known as total parenteral nutrition, or TPN) is reserved for use when the gut is not functioning adequately, for example in severe pancreatitis, or where gut rest is required. Nutrients and fluids are delivered via a central line into the bloodstream. This is rarely used for clients with dysphagia unless it coexists with a gastrointestinal problem. High rates of infection and other complications are associated with this form of non-oral feeding.

The effect of alternative feeding on a client's emotional and physical well-being has only recently been studied critically. In general, however, clients tend to tolerate PEGs better than NGs (that is, they are pulled out less frequently by clients).

The effects of an NG tube on swallowing and overall feeling of well-being

A fine-bore NG tube has long been considered to reduce the sensitivity of the gag reflex. As a result, while it will not impede the swallow of dysphagic clients – should a problem with reflux or vomiting occur, which is not uncommon in tube-fed individuals – the risk of aspiration increases significantly. For further information on the role of the gag reflex and aspiration, see Chapters 1 and 2.

Huggins *et al* (1999) identified potential benefits of NG tubes for the pharyngeal stage swallowing skills of clients with dysphagia, although their research was conducted on normal healthy adults. The most significant trends observed were an increase in oral to pharyngeal-stage transition values (hyolaryngeal excursion occurring earlier), longer duration of UES (cricopharyngeus) opening (which, in combination with the former, results in longer pharyngeal stage duration), and an increased delay in pharyngeal transit. In our opinion, however, these results should be viewed cautiously, and fuller investigation is required.

Onslow (1999), a speech and language therapist, detailed her experiences as a relatively long-term NG tube user, with a normal swallow. She reported the discomfort of

◆ Eating with the tube in situ, and the sensation that each swallow dragged it down
◆ Moving her head spontaneously to the left to talk to others, causing a strong swallow
◆ Tube flushing with room temperature water (between feeds)
◆ A full bladder caused by up to two litres of fluid per day

The effects of a PEG on swallowing

Long-term use of PEGs is increasing. Clinical experience indicates that many older clients (75 years plus) require a substantial period of time using PEG feeding and nil orally, before they are ready to benefit from rehabilitation of their swallow. This may be due to the prolonged effect of poor nutrition prior to, and immediately after, the neurological event. This may take over six months from the time of the neurological insult and, even in those with progressive diseases, improved nutrition and hydration appear to have a positive impact on swallowing skills. Part or full oral intake may then be resumed safely. The factors influencing these findings require further research.

Fluids

Fluids, without significant nutrition, may be administered via an intravenous infusion (IV), or subcutaneously (sub-cut fluids). Providing hydration in this way offers the advantage of determining whether a client's swallowing difficulties are due to a specific neurological cause, or can be attributed largely to dehydration, without committing to an NG tube which, ethically, it may not be appropriate to discontinue if there is no improvement in a client's condition.

IV fluids are administered via a vein. The site of entry is normally used for a maximum of 72 hours, although an IV can remain in situ for as long as necessary. The quantity of fluid given varies according to the acuteness of the underlying problem, three to four litres being administered over a 24-hour period.

Sub cutaneous (sub-cut) fluids, slowly administered under the skin, are a short-term measure, normally used as a last resort to rehydrate a client (usually only one litre), alongside oral hydration whenever possible.

If the client requires thickened fluids to reduce the risk of aspiration, a starch-based thickening agent (as opposed to a gum-based product) will release the liquid, ensuring adequate hydration if sufficient quantities of fluid are ingested.

Transitional feeding

A hierarchy of intake routes, nutrition intake and fluid intake is provided below (see Table 9.1). The three areas should always be considered together. The aim should be to maintain a client's optimal nutrition and hydration status as detailed in the centre and right-hand columns, irrespective of their swallowing skills.

Table 9.1 Transitional Feeding

Nil by any route	no nutritional intake	no fluid intake, very severe risk of dehydration
↓ ↑	↓ ↑	↓ ↑
IV or sub-cut fluids	a few mouthfuls each meal	2 cups taken per day, risk of dehydration
↓ ↑	↓ ↑	↓ ↑
Gastrostomy/NG tube feeding (including tastes for pleasure)	half meal eaten, but not on a regular basis, and not a well-balanced intake	4 cups taken per day, client needs encouragement
↓ ↑	↓ ↑	↓ ↑
Oral plus gastrostomy/NG tube feeding to meet nutritional needs	half meal eaten regularly, involving a variety of foods	6 cups taken per day
↓ ↑	↓ ↑	↓ ↑
Oral	nutritional needs fully met	hydration needs met, taking 8 cups plus per day

Strategies

No dysphagia management plan would be complete without advice regarding strategies for safe oral intake, whether as part of a wholly oral route or as part of a transitional feeding programme.

Small, frequent meals are generally the most acceptable and appetising, particularly for those with depressed appetites. Some clients find thermal crockery, which maintains the temperature of the food (normally suitable for both cold and hot foods) of great value.

Dietary texture modification ought not to result in less appetising portions. Clinicians must be aware of menu specifications available within their care settings (for example, soft easy-chew, purée and very soft diet) and, wherever possible, match their recommendations to these options. Involving clients in selecting foods from the menu can increase compliance. Cultural preferences must be respected.

We suggest avoiding purée whenever possible. Very few clients really require purée – other than those who experience difficulty inhibiting chewing, such as some clients with cognitive changes and those with a severe delay in laryngeal closure. The nutritional content of purée may be reduced following the addition of water to produce the appropriate texture, and clients rarely eat sufficient quantities. Puréed food can result in reduced sensation compared with soft foods. Unfortunately, at times, care staff find that the foods provided as soft, moist options are unsuitable and only purée is available at that sitting. It is often difficult to determine the origins of purée, and care staff may be tempted to mix different tastes together. Representatives of suppliers of fluid thickening agents can provide demonstrations to catering staff, showing techniques for making food more appetising using thickening powder in purée, which is placed in moulds that resemble the original food (for example, pork chops, carrots). Also, they can demonstrate techniques for soaking foods such as cakes and biscuits, which softens them into a smooth consistency, removing their inappropriate crumbly texture. Baby food is not nutritionally complete for adults. At the time of writing, some suppliers in the

United Kingdom are introducing frozen puréed meals. These are nutritionally complete and maintain their form when on a plate.

Medication

Difficulty swallowing tablets may be a common reason for referral to the speech and language therapy team, necessitating close liaison with the pharmacy department. Elixirs and medications that can be given via suspension may easily overcome such problems. Some commonly used medications will disperse in water given sufficient time, but may be chalky and therefore remain difficult to swallow. Crushing tablets or opening capsules should require care and a full Control of Substances Hazardous to Health (COSHH) assessment (see Chapter 11). Krawczk and Codling (1998) suggested the use of stickers for drug charts to alert the medical and pharmacy teams to potential swallowing difficulties.

UTENSILS

The provision and use of appropriate utensils can significantly enhance the pleasure and safety of eating and drinking. Self-feeding is preferred as it encourages normalisation and reduces the risk of aspiration. Altering traditional practices, particularly within inpatient units may, however, prove to be a long-term (years-long) process.

Foods

The aim is to use normal utensils wherever possible. Teaspoons are popular, offering a suitable, controllable quantity of food. Alternatively, select dessertspoons that are narrower at the front and relatively flat, to provide a slightly larger mouthful for those who require a larger bolus. Metal spoons provide normal kinaesthetic feedback to the client. If there is concern regarding a bite reflex, this should be dealt with first, rather than opting for plastic or bone spoons (see Chapter 6, 'Oral Stage Management').

Forks, if used with care, are acceptable, and are the preferred option for savoury courses. In addition they are difficult to overfill. It is advisable to specify how full the spoon or fork should be.

Drinks

Ideally, drinks should be taken from a normal cup or glass, with or without supported or hand-on-hand feeding. To prevent the client tilting their head backwards once the first third has been drunk, the contents of the cup can be topped up as required. Alternative cups include 'flexicups' (flexible and lightweight, shaped to facilitate drinking without having to tilt the head back) and a 'dysphagia cup' (shaped to allow sufficient nose clearance, and to permit cup contents to flow into the centre of the mouth; weighted with a large handle). See Appendix II for suppliers.

We suggest that spouted cups be avoided. It is difficult to monitor the quantity of fluid being given; they encourage a head-back position and feeding in a supine position, which can lead to aspiration; they encourage a primitive sucking pattern; they are plastic, therefore providing feedback unlike that from a normal cup; and they are difficult to keep clean. The same arguments apply to baby feeder cups, which can also infantilise the adult.

Straws promote independence and control. 'Pat Saunders straws' (see Appendix II) contain one-way valves to ensure that a drink does not fall back down the straw once sucking ceases. This prevents excess ingestion of air and can reduce fatigue. The straws are made of rigid plastic, do not bend easily and initially require a strong suck to pull the fluid up the straw. Alternatively, normal flexible straws with a moderate diameter can be cut down to one-half to two-thirds of their length.

Offering fluids on a spoon also promotes safety and independence. We do not recommend syringing fluids into the client's mouth, as this reduces oral control and the bolus may overspill the base of the tongue into the airway before the swallow is fully triggered. If care staff feel that they are unable to cease this practice, it may be possible to negotiate standards on the ways that syringes are used. Examples of such guidelines may include restricting their use to small doses of controlled medication only; avoiding their use with clients with low levels of alertness or those who will not open their mouth; permitting only trained staff to use syringes in this manner, and providing a maximum of 2ml at any one time while observing and feeling for a swallow.

INTRODUCTION

This chapter is based on the two Royal College of Speech and Language Therapists publications (RCSLT, 1996 Chapters 4 and 6; 1998a, Chapter 2). They are essential reading for anyone working in this area. The clinician must take responsibility for being fully informed.

This chapter will cover the following:

- Local dysphagia policy
- Referral
- Assessment
- Intervention
- Discharge
- Safety procedures
- Legal issues
- Other issues to consider

LOCAL DYSPHAGIA POLICY

It is essential that the clinician's job description includes the assessment and management of dysphagia. If it has not been mentioned, they are not legally covered by their employing agency to carry out this type of work. The speech and language therapy service will formulate and publish a local dysphagia policy that will be available to all interested parties. The local policy needs to include clear reporting and documentation procedures, as well as advice on how to proceed in the event of a dispute about client management. Clinicians may find it helpful to involve the local clinical risk coordinator for the employing agency in formulating an effective risk management strategy for aspiration, together with other members of the multidisciplinary team. It is important for the clinician to be familiar with the contents of the local dysphagia policy.

The RCSLT advises that written information about the service is to be available to other health service staff, other agencies and users. We suggest that client information leaflets about the service in general (including the clinician's name) and videofluoroscopy are made available. In addition, information for clients and carers from voluntary and support organisations will be given, such as the Motor Neurone Disease Association, Headway.

With regard to videofluoroscopy and FEESS, 'The speech and language therapist must ensure that approval has been given by the employing authority or directorate, with recognition of competence to perform the procedure[s], adherence to local Health and Safety Policies and adequate professional liability insurance cover, either through the Trust, the Professional Body or Professional Union' (RCSLT, 1999).

It is unusual for speech and language therapists in the United Kingdom to perform suction (see Chapter 8, 'Tracheostomies and Ventilators'). Reilly and Carroll (1992) state that, if a clinician is to carry out suction, 'they should be certain it is included in their job description and is part of their district dysphagia policy ... If training is not available then we would suggest that therapists seriously consider the legal implications of undertaking this duty'.

REFERRAL

At the time of writing, to gain access, a client requires a written referral from the medical practitioner responsible for their care. This should indicate clearly that the reason for referral is for dysphagia evaluation and management. Where the clinician identifies a suspected swallowing problem – for example in a client who is referred for assessment and management of communication difficulties – a written referral should be requested before assessing the swallowing problem.

Inpatients referred for assessments should be seen within two working days of receiving the referral. Urgent or acute outpatient and community referrals are seen within two weeks. Non-urgent outpatient and community referrals are seen within four weeks. Liaison with the members of the multidisciplinary team, or with the carer, is advisable to clarify the urgency of the referral, and to obtain maximum information prior to the assessment. Domiciliary visits need to follow appropriate safety and 'duty of care' guidelines.

ASSESSMENT

The clinician needs to function as part of many multidisciplinary teams, having a clear understanding of the roles of the other professionals. We suggest close liaison, and that joint assessments be undertaken where appropriate. The clinician will use a variety of methods, such as case history, observation and investigative techniques. If a client has a tracheostomy and/or is ventilator-dependent, the clinician is responsible for acquainting herself with the different types of tracheostomy tubes, and understanding the implications for assessment and management.

'Where a client is already taking some food or drink orally, the clinician should observe them doing so. Where the client is being fed non-orally, the team should be consulted before trial swallows are attempted' (RCSLT, 1996). This is because some clients may be on gut rest: for example, those with severe pancreatitis. The results, including the amounts given, should be fully documented in the clinician's notes and, for inpatients, in the medical and nursing notes.

The clinician should be involved in the decision to recommend further investigations of dysphagia, for example videofluoroscopy or fibre-optic endoscopic evaluation of swallowing safety, in order to plan intervention effectively. Clinicians should not undertake a programme of intervention if there is insufficient information about the swallowing anatomy and physiology. The responsible physician should be informed, if this is the case. The results of the investigations, assessments and planned management will be discussed with client and carer. We suggest that the clinician records in writing that this discussion has taken place.

INTERVENTION

All forms of intervention will be discussed with the team, client and carer before commencing, and a written care plan formulated. The clinician will document any change in the client's management in the clinician's, medical and nursing notes. Written guidelines relating to feeding and other related interventions are given to the client and carers where appropriate (see examples in Appendix IV). If broad agreement exists between the clinician, client, carer and multidisciplinary team, the management plan may proceed. If disagreement exists, every effort should be made to resolve it through discussion, as it is important to have full cooperation if the management is to be effective. If the client or carer refuses to consent to the planned intervention, this should be documented and communicated to the physician responsible for the client's care.

If disagreement exists among the team, particularly between the doctor responsible for the client's care and other team members, every effort should be made to resolve it through discussion. If the doctor chooses a course of action contrary to the advice of the clinician, and the clinician believes such action may be inappropriate or may cause the client harm, the clinician is advised to record their opinion in writing to the doctor, and the clinician's manager will be informed. In some cases it may be necessary to withdraw involvement.

The clinician may delegate certain therapy tasks to other team members, the client or carer. These may include feeding and supervision of oral intake. The clinician remains responsible for the proxy intervention, even when another delegated person carries it out, provided that the written instructions are followed correctly.

Clients will need to be reviewed to ensure that progress has been maintained; to evaluate their readiness for intervention, and to monitor any change in status. The frequency of review should be considered carefully. Clients with degenerative disorders may need regular review over many months.

DISCHARGE

The clinician will decide if and when discharge is indicated, in full consultation with the team, client and carer. A written summary of the outcome of the intervention will be distributed to the appropriate people involved. Changes in the client's condition or environment may result in a further period of intervention at a later stage. The process for re-referral and for reaching the clinician should specific questions or concerns arise will be made clear to the client, carer and family doctor (see example in Appendix IV).

SAFETY PROCEDURES

The clinician will adhere to local policies regarding health and safety, such as cross-infection or suction (see also Chapter 11 'Health and Safety'; RCSLT, 1996, 1999). Due consideration needs to be given to the safety of providing therapy in an environment without medical support. This is best discussed fully with medical staff prior to intervention. In addition, the domiciliary clinician needs to consider their own personal safety.

LEGAL ISSUES

Documentation

The RCSLT Guidelines for endoscopic evaluation of the vocal tract and radiological imaging (1999) can be applied equally to all areas of working with clients with dysphagia. They include the following suggestions:

◆ Departmental records should include all the client's referral details, along with any assessments, letters and reports.

◆ Every contact should be recorded, dated and signed.

◆ The results of any additional investigation, such as a videofluoroscopy or FEESS, including any untoward occurrences, complications or emergencies and how they were managed, must be written in the client's medical records. Any adverse incident needs to be reported according to the local policies and procedures.

◆ Recorded material is part of the client's records and so must be kept according to local policies. A system needs to be in place that maintains confidentiality.

We advise writing legibly, in black pen, in case the clinician's notes need to be photocopied for litigation purposes.

Legal liability

The employing authority is vicariously liable for the clinician within the scope of their duties; that is, it will support the clinician in litigation, provided the charge is not criminal. However, the support depends on whether the clinician was performing duties covered in their job description. Registered members of RCSLT who have paid the requisite subscription have professional indemnity insurance that specifically cites dysphagia as an area of work. 'Whenever a member is aware of circumstances likely to give rise to a claim, immediate notice must be given to the Professional Director at the College Offices. No liability must be admitted, no admission, arrangement or promise of payment made' (RCSLT *Practice Register and Directory*, 2000).

Decision-making

Primary responsibility for taking decisions which could bring about a new 'life-threatening' situation rests with the medical practitioner concerned. Rice (1999) states: 'the doctor is responsible for decisions to withhold, give or withdraw medical treatment: in law, fluid given by tube is regarded as a medical treatment'. The views of the multidisciplinary team should be considered and should be based on ethical reasoning and not driven by emotion. The aim of care is dependent on the diagnosis and prognosis. It may be to prolong life or to offer comfort during the process of dying. 'A professional carer has a duty to prolong life but not to inappropriately prolong dying' (Lennard-Jones, 1998).

Informed medical consent and client competence

Consent should be recorded in the clinician's notes. The RCSLT Legal Pack (1998b) quotes Judge Gordon Ashton, who writes in the *Elderly Care Handbook*:

'It is illegal for people who are judged to have mental capacity, not to be enabled to give informed medical consent to procedures. Competence is presumed unless the contrary is proved and means that the patient has:

◆ Sufficient understanding and intelligence to comprehend the nature, purpose and likely purpose of treatment and the consequences of undergoing or refusing treatment

◆ The ability to communicate his decision in relation to the particular treatment.'

If the client refuses to participate in the clinician's proposed management, this should be documented in the records. The clinician will ensure that the client understands the consequences of refusal to participate before discharging the client.

Treatment without an incompetent adult's consent is legal in emergencies, in order to provide treatment to save the life of an unconscious individual, or where treatment is considered by the physician to be in the best interest of the client who is mentally incapable of giving consent.

Advanced directives and living wills

'A living will is made to request that certain treatment should or should not be given in certain situations if the individual becomes incompetent and unable to participate in decisions that affect him/her' (RCSLT, 1998b). At the time of writing, advanced directives and living wills are not subject to legislation, although there have been some cases that appear to support them (see Chapter 12). The *Legal Pack* goes on to state:

'It is assumed that a speech and language therapist would only be involved in the presence of a solicitor or other professionals, to establish competence and enable the client to complete the document at his/her request. The therapist is not advised to act as a witness to the signature, unless satisfied as to the person's competence to make a living will. Similarly, as yet there is no legislation whereby someone may delegate the power to make decisions about treatment for another person.'

Duty of care

This occurs from the moment the clinician sees the client, and not from the date of referral. It continues until the clinician closes the case. Duty can only be determined on the basis of what most clinicians would do, not on the instructions of a member of another profession, no matter how senior they may be (Horner, 1999). Negligence is a breach of a duty of care. It can be an act or omission that causes harm resulting in damage to the client. Clinicians remain responsible at all times for their own acts and omissions. Clinicians are expected to conform to the standard of a reasonable practitioner. The nature of dysphagia may mean that the clinician is required to assess or review a client at short notice; therefore clinicians need to be available to discharge their duty of care according to local guidelines.

Horner (1999) provides an example of the dilemma where a hospital consultant refuses to refer clients with dysphagia to speech and language therapists. In it, the clinician notices that while working with a client with a disorder of communication the client is experiencing swallowing difficulties. The clinician is concerned for the client's safety and for their own responsibility under the common law duty of care. Horner suggests that the issue be dealt with in the following manner.

- The most senior therapist within the organisation must meet the consultant and explain that, while their opinions are respected though not agreed with, their right to decide how their patients are to be treated is fully accepted, and that speech and language therapists also have a legal duty of care. This duty is determined on the basis of what most speech and language therapists would do, not on the instructions of a member of another profession.
- The senior therapist will inform the consultant that the speech and language therapy service will not perform any more dysphagia assessments on any of the consultant's patients until they is prepared to vary their present instruction. The therapists will not have any professional relationship with these patients and therefore no duty of care. This is because 'it is impossible for a professional therapist to treat one condition but ignore a potentially more serious one'.
- The consultant will be informed that the therapist will explain the situation to the next of kin should they enquire about the reasons for this decision.
- The senior clinician will confirm in writing to the consultant what was discussed in this meeting and will copy the letter to the chief executive of the trust.
- Next, the issue may be raised with the trust managers, perhaps through the medical director or the senior health professional with responsibility for clinical governance.
- If the issue is not treated with sufficient seriousness, then perhaps the matter will be taken higher, to the chief executive or the chair of the trust.
- Finally, all the speech and language therapists within the service should be informed of the action they must take as individuals, so as to protect themselves from an accusation of failure in their duty of care.

◆ Should a member of the staff disobey this explicit instruction (perhaps because of an unfortunate interpretation of their ethical duty of care) the manager of the service must start disciplinary proceedings.

In conclusion, Horner recognises that this action may destroy the professional relationships in the team, but 'the consequences of ignoring such a situation are equally serious, for the individual therapist and for the whole organisation'.

Duty to act

If difficulties arise in a life-threatening situation and a positive duty to act arises, the clinician is required to do whatever would be reasonably expected. For instance, Reilly and Carroll (1992) state that 'Although suction is not generally recognised as within the scope of a speech therapist's duties, in special circumstances it may be appropriate.' An example of this might be that, if a client's airway is compromised through aspiration and a coincidental event such as an epileptic fit occurs simultaneously, the priority is to maintain the safety of the client's airway. Clinicians need to follow the local health and safety guidelines and be adequately prepared: for example by attending cardiopulmonary resuscitation training.

OTHER ISSUES TO CONSIDER

Competence

Clinicians have varying degrees of experience. There may be certain situations where a clinician recognises that an intervention should be carried out by a clinician with greater experience, or a referral should be made to a specialist from another discipline. Failure to recognise such situations may amount to a breach of duty of care. Issues relating to clients who are competent and those who are unable to make an autonomous decision are discussed in Chapter 12, 'Making Ethical Decisions'.

Skill mix

At the time of writing, training in the assessment and management of dysphagia is being incorporated into undergraduate and postgraduate degree courses and postgraduate diplomas. Previously, clinicians have received a post-basic level training, approximately six months after qualifying. It is important that clinicians can refer to colleagues with specific responsibilities for dysphagia and to secure a specialist opinion. It is advisable for clinicians to be members of appropriate RCSLT specific interest groups. Continued professional development should be available to all staff and relevant courses may be identified in conjunction with the clinician's manager or supervisor, according to need. If a clinician is not trained to an advanced level, they must gain their clinical experience in a supervised setting.

Assistants: speech and language therapy assistants, healthcare assistants and general assistants

Assistants may undertake elements of swallowing therapy that the clinician feels able to delegate to carers – for example, thermal stimulation. It is the clinician's responsibility to train adequately assistants, nursing staff, volunteers or carers in the task required and the necessary safety procedures (see Chapter 11). Chapter 5, 'General Issues in Management', provides further details on the role and responsibilities of nurses in the management of dysphagia.

Confidentiality

Clinicians in the UK need to be aware of the Data Protection Act 1998, the European Directive for Data Protection 1988, The Computer Misuse Act 1990 and the Access to Medical Records Act 1990. Professionals must guard against accidental or unintentional breaches of confidentiality by not leaving client's files out and asking leading questions in front of others, particularly with reference to HIV status.

Chapter 11: Health and Safety

INTRODUCTION

Each clinician has a legal duty to be fully informed of and to adhere to their local policies in order to safeguard themselves, their clients, colleagues, students and visitors. The content of this chapter relates to the authors' experience of good practice, and it is suggested that clinicians note that practice may vary depending on local policies; therefore it is imperative always to refer to these local policies. Appropriate and regular training is advised in these areas. (See 'A Strategy For Service Management – Health and Safety At Work', RCSLT, 1996.)

LOCAL HEALTH AND SAFETY POLICY

The UK Health and Safety at Work Act 1974 details the requirements of the clinician. Each department will have its own local health and safety policy that needs to be updated regularly. Key personnel who can advise clinicians include the following:

◆ Health and safety advisor – each department is usually required to have a representative for liaison with the local health and safety advisor. This is often a speech and language therapist with management responsibility.

◆ Occupational health physician.

◆ Infection control nurse.

◆ Radiation protection advisor.

◆ Patient-handling nurse, or other suitably trained staff, such as a physiotherapist.

OCCUPATIONAL HEALTH

Clinicians need to ensure their immunisations are up to date, particularly Hepatitis B, TB, polio, rubella and tetanus.

Hepatitis B virus (HBV)

The symptoms of this are general malaise, reduced appetite, weight loss and jaundice, which can result in liver disease that can be fatal. It is transferred by blood and other body fluids including sputum, saliva, nasal secretions, tears, vomitus and sweat. It takes three to six months for symptoms to develop. Coughing, sneezing, sharing eating or sharing drinking utensils cannot transfer it, but sharing razors and toothbrushes can. Immunisation may last for up to five years and involves a series of three injections. It is safe to be immunised during pregnancy. HBV is very much more infectious than the human immunodeficiency virus and may lead to serious complications.

Human immunodeficiency virus (HIV)

The virus has been detected in blood and other body fluids including sputum, saliva, nasal secretions, tears, vomitus and sweat (Larsen, 1998). Larsen states that occupational exposure through the skin or mucous membrane to skin contact has been reported but is extremely rare. The majority of occupational exposures occur through needle-stick injuries, where the instrument has come into contact with HIV-infected body fluids, such as blood. However, the risk of transmission is still considered extremely low.

INFECTION CONTROL

Universal precautions

The healthy body is able to defend itself against transient pathogenic organisms in most individuals. However, the ill client has an increased risk of cross infection transmitted by hand (Gilmour & Hughes, 1997). Often we are not aware that a client, carer, student or colleague is potentially infected with diseases including HBV or HIV. Similarly, clinicians may be unaware that they are infected. Therefore, universal precautions are used to protect the clinician from the client and vice versa. The American Centres for Disease Control and Prevention recommend that all professionals consider all their clients as potentially infected with blood-borne viruses and pathogens. This ensures the use of the same precautions with everyone. University College London Hospitals (1997) and Larsen (1998) recommend the following:

◆ Cover all cuts and abrasions on skin with a waterproof occlusive dressing. Clinicians with non-intact skin as a result of dermatitis or cuts should refrain from touching the client directly without gloves on.

- Disposable examination gloves must be worn when touching body fluids, mucous membranes or non-intact skin of clients (for example, when assessing for increased oral tone and hypersensitivity); when handling surfaces soiled with such fluids; when performing invasive procedures (for example, a FEESS), or handling components of tracheostomy tubes.
- Goggles, visors or facemasks must be available and should be worn by staff when contact with body products is expected or anticipated.
- Care must be taken to clean and disinfect any equipment according to local policies.

NB Some individuals may be allergic to latex. If an allergy develops, it can result in anaphylactic shock, which is a serious allergic hypersensitive reaction of the body to a foreign substance. This can lead to death if emergency medical treatment is not given.

Infection control is particularly important as the incidence of antibiotic resistant pathogens in healthcare settings increases. These can seriously impair the client's health. The costs are great in terms of drug treatment and may require an increase in length of stay in hospital. An example of one of these infections is multi-resistant staphylococcus aureus (MRSA). Also included are other micro-organisms that may be found in healthcare settings, such as clostridium difficile, rota virus, klebsiella, campylobacter and salmonella.

Features of good practice

- Keep nails short.
- Do not wear nail varnish.
- It is advisable to have one's own personal tube of hand cream. Do not use multi-dose pots of cream, as these may become contaminated.
- Long hair must be tied back.
- Necklaces must be tucked inside clothing.
- Personal clothing should be laundered regularly.
- Bars of soap must not be communal. Use the wall-mounted liquid soap supplied.
- Domiciliary clinicians should take alcohol rubs, gels or liquid soap in containers on home visits.

- Wipe torches and stethoscopes with alcohol wipes between clients.
- Pat Saunders straws should be single-client issue and cleaned with hot water and detergent.
- Laryngeal mirrors for thermal stimulation must be sent to the central sterile supplies department for autoclaving.

Hand washing (based on UCLH Infection Control Policy, 1997)

Gilmour and Hughes (1997) suggest that this is still a neglected practice in the clinical area. Many studies demonstrate that it is the single most important way of reducing cross infection. During clinical work, sleeves should be rolled up above the elbows and wrist watches, other wrist jewellery and rings should be removed. The rationale behind this is that thorough clinical hand washing cannot take place when these are worn. Plain wedding bands are acceptable as they harbour fewer pathogens than those with stones or engravings. If unable to remove rings, wash and dry very thoroughly around and under them.

Hand washing is required between each client contact. An alcohol rub can be used in place of hand washing when a sink is not close to hand and the hands are not soiled. If a hand rub is used, it must be thoroughly distributed over all the surfaces of the hands and wrists, paying close attention to the fingertips and thumbs. Gloved hands must always be washed following removal of gloves.

The procedure for hand washing is as follows:

- Roll up sleeves and remove wrist watch and rings.
- Use running hot water.
- Wet hands and apply one to two pumps of liquid soap or antiseptic into the palm of your hand.
- Hold hands down below elbow height to prevent water running on to forearms.
- Rub the hands vigorously to lather all surfaces of the hands and wrists, paying particular attention to the thumbs, fingertips and finger webs.
- Rinse the hands and wrists well, removing all the soap.
- Turn off the water using elbows or wrists on elbow taps.

◆ Pat the hands and wrists thoroughly to dry, using paper towels.

◆ If elbow taps are not present, first dry the hands thoroughly, then turn off the taps using a fresh paper towel.

◆ Dispose of the paper towel by using the foot-operated pedal bin. Do not use hands to lift the bin lid as they will become recontaminated.

Source isolation procedure

Before entering a source isolation room:

◆ Read the notice on the door

◆ Remove white coats or outside clothing (preferably leaving these on a hook outside the room)

◆ Remove wrist watch

◆ Put on a yellow apron and disposable gloves

Inside the room:

◆ Do not touch the client or anything else unnecessarily

◆ Do not sit on the bed

◆ When leaving the room take off the apron, followed by the gloves

◆ Discard the apron and gloves in the bin in the client's room

◆ Wash and dry hands thoroughly

Equipment:

◆ Items may be brought out of the room, but they must be cleaned and disinfected according to the disinfection policy, or disposed of appropriately;

◆ Ordinary cutlery and crockery can be used, which is processed in the normal way. Left-over food may remain on the client's tray and is disposed of in the hospital or ward kitchen.

If the clinician is concerned about a hand lesion, skin problems associated with hand washing, transmission of any infection or exposure, it is suggested that the local infection control or occupational health departments be contacted for advice. Clinicians with eczema are at high risk of acquiring resistant hospital-associated staphylococci.

FOOD SAFETY (from Food Hygiene Policy, Camden and Islington Community Health Services NHS Trust, 1999)

The number of reported confirmed cases of food poisoning continues to rise every year. Hygienic preparation and serving of food is paramount. Contamination of food with pathogens, poor temperature control and inadequate cooking remain major risks. To reduce these risks, new laws have been introduced: Food Safety (General Food Hygiene) Regulations 1995, Food Safety (Temperature Control) Regulations 1995, Food Labelling Regulations 1996 and Food Labelling (Amendment) Regulations (1998.)

The first document outlines various levels of training required for food storage, preparation, cooking, handling and service. Clinicians need to be aware of the regulations that specify statutory minimum and maximum temperatures for storage. This is to reduce the growth of bacteria to as low a level as possible (hot food must be held at temperatures exceeding 63°C, food in refrigerators must be stored between 0 and 5 °C, and ice-cream at –10°C). Room temperature is ideal for bacterial growth; therefore food should not be left at this temperature. In a hospital, unopened food may remain in the refrigerator until its expiry date. However, once opened, food may remain in there for only 24 hours and must be labelled with the client's name and the date of opening. After this, it must be disposed of promptly. Basic food hygiene principles apply to the contents of a fridge: for example, cooked and uncooked food not sharing the same shelf. We suggest that clinicians refer to local food hygiene policies.

Ice cubes

Freezers can allow pathogens including xanthomonas maltophilia to develop in ice cubes and trays. It is recommended that drinking-quality water be used in freshly cleaned containers, or preferably disposable ice cube bags (available from supermarkets) should be used. If made in a freezer compartment, they need to be renewed every week.

PATIENT HANDLING

Clinicians must be aware of the importance of back care and consider both their personal safety and that of the client if assisting with positioning of the client for assessment or intervention. We suggest asking nurses, physiotherapists, occupational therapists or other suitably trained staff to position patients.

WHAT TO DO IF A CLIENT CHOKES

If a client chokes on food the main aim of first aid is to get them to cough up the obstruction, or for the clinician to remove it with their fingers. Local procedures will vary. Camden and Islington Community Health Services NHS Trust recommends the following:

- Try to get the client to cough up the obstruction by hitting them firmly between the shoulder blades with the heel of your hand. Do this up to five times.
- If this does not work, stand behind them, putting both arms around their waist.
- Find the area which is about 2–3cm above their navel.
- Clench one fist, with your thumb towards the person and wrap your other hand around the clenched fist.
- Using short, firm actions, press inwards and upwards. Do this up to five times.
- If that does not work, try looking inside their mouth for an obstruction. If there is one, try hooking it out with your fingers, but stop immediately if there is any risk of pushing it further in, or if the client shows signs of biting down.
- If that does not work, get the client to bend over so that their head is lower than their chest. Repeat the firm hits between the shoulder blades and the abdominal thrusts if necessary. Do not perform this manoeuvre on pregnant women, obese clients or children under four years of age.

The RCSLT guidelines for endoscopic evaluation of the vocal tract and radiological imaging (1999) recommend that speech and language therapists consider first aid and resuscitation training if participating in invasive procedures.

THE CONTROL OF SUBSTANCES HAZARDOUS TO HEALTH (COSHH)
REGULATIONS (1989) AND FEESS

COSHH regulations are designed to safeguard people who work with substances that have the potential to harm. Of relevance to clinicians is Glutaraldehyde, a highly noxious disinfectant solution for cleaning fibre-optic nasendoscopes used in FEESS. The nasendoscope must receive high-level decontamination, if not sterilisation, by an appropriately trained person who is registered in the use of the procedure. We suggest the clinician refers to the local infection control policy.

In addition, universal precautions will be used when performing a FEESS to prevent disease transmission via contact with the equipment and cross-infection of both clients and staff involved. The clinician must be familiar with the indications and contraindications, as well as possible drug interaction of topical anaesthetics and nasal decongestants.

WASTE

Under the Environmental Protection Act 1990, the Health and Safety at Work Act 1974 and the Control of Waste Regulation 1992, clinicians are responsible for ensuring that waste is disposed of safely. The following procedures are common:

◆ Domestic or household waste such as kitchen waste, dead flowers, newspapers or office waste, is placed in black sacks.
◆ Clinical waste such as sputum-soiled wipes and equipment used for oral hygiene are placed in yellow sacks.
◆ Small fragments of glass and sharp objects are disposed of into rigid disposable containers. Large or whole glass may be disposed of either into rigid plastic containers or wrapped in paper before placing in cardboard boxes and appropriately labelled 'Danger! Glass!'
◆ Special waste, such as unused barium, should not be disposed of down a sink as it can set solid in the soil pipes.

RADIATION PROTECTION AND VIDEOFLUOROSCOPY

The radiologist has 'overall responsibility for the procedure and together with the radiographer, is responsible for monitoring ionising radiation exposure ... This investigation should only be performed in a specially designed screening room within the x-ray department with access to medical and nursing personnel, sterilisation and emergency equipment. Ideally, it should be performed within a multidisciplinary environment' (RSCLT guidelines for speech and language therapists, 1999.)

At the time of writing, new legislation is being prepared regarding radiation regulations. The main principles are of justification, optimisation and limitation. First, can the clinician justify the use of radiation? Will the benefit to the client be more than the detriment of risk? Usually it is the radiologist who has the final responsibility to make a decision to proceed with the investigation. Optimisation refers to using the lowest possible amount of radiation to establish the information the clinician requires for a diagnosis. Limitation refers to maximum radiation doses that can be received by staff or members of the public. Exposures for medical purposes are not subject to limits.

Doses to staff can be reduced by minimising exposure time, increasing distance from the radiation and by use of shielding. The person operating the X-ray equipment is responsible for the healthcare worker's safety, and staff should always follow their direction. If the clinician does not need to be close to the client, they should stand as far back as possible while the X-ray beam is on, preferably behind a shielded screen. (If X-rays are performed on wards, follow the lead of other staff and stand well away when called to do so.) If the clinician remains close to the client, the professional should wear the protective clothing provided. Bear in mind that lead aprons, thyroid shields and gloves are designed only to protect against radiation scattered from the client. The clinician must never allow any part of their body to enter the primary X-ray beam. If the clinician is given one or more personal dosemeters they should be worn as directed and submitted promptly for reading. Appropriate universal infection control measures should be used in line with local policies, for example assessing clients who are MRSA positive last, in order that the room and equipment can be cleaned adequately.

The clinician needs to be familiar with the preparation of materials to be used, such as the strength of the barium, making an appropriate decision about whether to use Omnipaque and the avoidance of barium and Gastrograffin where there is a risk of aspiration, food preparation and hygiene procedures.

It is recommended that clinicians attend training by the radiation protection advisor for their unit and discuss issues, such as performing videofluoroscopy if pregnant, with the superintendent radiographer.

Finally, if clinicians do not know about any of these policies, it is important that they take responsibility themselves to obtain copies of them and find out more from the appropriately trained staff.

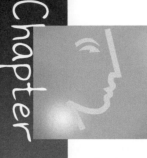

Chapter 12: Making Ethical Decisions

INTRODUCTION

'Speech and language therapists' role in the care of people with swallowing difficulties is increasingly recognised and advances in medical science are leading to more people surviving with multiple, complex diagnoses. These factors are likely to lead to speech and language therapists contributing increasingly to difficult decisions concerning their future care and management. To do so effectively we need to be knowledgeable about ethics and the guidance available, and to apply ethical principles.' (Rice, 1999)

This chapter will focus on the following areas:

◆ Definitions of ethical values

◆ Ethical decision-making

◆ Living wills and advanced directives

◆ The effects of dehydration and starvation on the client who is dying

◆ Alternative feeding as a treatment

◆ Guidelines for gastrostomy tube placement

We advise that clinicians be familiar with the Code of Ethics and Professional Conduct section in *Communicating Quality 2* (RCSLT, 1996).

DEFINITIONS OF ETHICAL VALUES (From Pannbacker *et al*, 1996)

Autonomy

Autonomy is a commitment to respect an individual's independent actions and choices; it includes the client's dignity, worth and rights. Possibly the most important member of the team is the client, as ultimately they decide whether to follow the professionals' recommendations for management.

Beneficence

Beneficence is the obligation to act in the best interest of the client's welfare. This means that the clinician's intervention must be appropriate, needed and beneficial to the client and family. The client needs to be able to decide whether to commence intervention based on accurate information about the diagnosis, prognosis for improvement and the possible outcome of the intervention. 'Rehabilitation teams sometimes struggle with a perceived incompatibility between client autonomy and beneficence' (Pannbacker *et al*, 1996). For example, altering the client's goals because the team concludes that the decision is in the client's best interest is paternalistic but may be justified. To ensure beneficence, clinicians need (a) to make intervention personal to the individual client, (b) to delegate to other professional staff or carers only when appropriate, and (c) to maintain high standards of competence.

Harm avoidance (non-maleficence)

Harm avoidance is an obligation not to inflict evil, harm or risk of harm on others. Malpractice, as defined by Silverman (1992), is 'any type of negligent conduct by a professional that causes his or her patient to be harmed either physically or emotionally'. According to Rowland (1988), as quoted in Pannbacker *et al* (1996), malpractice includes the following:

◆ Misdiagnosis
◆ Failure to reveal alternative treatment
◆ Improper or sub-standard treatment
◆ Failure to refer when appropriate
◆ Referral to an inferior system for treatment
◆ Breach of an active contract for service or a product
◆ Breach of an implied contract
◆ Failure to instruct properly in the use of a potentially hazardous product
◆ Failure to warn of a potential hazard or harm

Justice

Justice is the 'equal distribution of benefits and burdens and fair allocation of scarce resources ... in the spirit of team work, professionals should be willing to help those who are carrying heavy workloads' (Pannbacker *et al*, 1996).

Confidentiality

Confidentiality is the understanding that any information divulged by the client to the clinician will not be revealed to another person, whether in verbal or written form, unless required to do so by law: for example, if the client reveals the intent to commit a crime.

Professional responsibility

Professional responsibility is an obligation to observe the rules of professional conduct with clients, colleagues and the community as a whole.

Truth

Truth refers to the disclosure of all pertinent information, including that which may reflect poorly on the informer. For example, clinicians are human and not infallible and may make an error that can affect the diagnosis or the results of the intervention. In this situation the client needs to be kept informed. The notion of truth also applies to making reasonable prognostic statements.

ETHICAL DECISION-MAKING

When clients are competent, 'they are the best judge of what represents an acceptable level of burden of risk' (BMA, 1999). According to Rice (1999), 'If a client who is "competent" refuses treatment there is no ethical dilemma and the refusal is a legal right (autonomy principle). However an ethical dilemma exists if the client is not able to be autonomous. The ethical principles of the process include beneficence, that is, the consideration of the benefits versus burdens (nonmaleficence) of the treatment.'

Johns (1993) reports that 'Central to effective professional practice are the contradictions between practitioners' espoused values and beliefs, usually articulated within a philosophy for practice, and the way they actually practise.' His paper demonstrates how effective ethical actions can be developed through guided reflection using shared experiences. It is suggested that this can be achieved by being client-centred, involving clients and families in intervention, giving and receiving feedback with other colleagues, and understanding the factors which cause the clinician stress and which limit their potential for intervention. Feelings play a significant role in ethical decision-making, that is, 'the knowledge of self and the impact of self on others and the impact of others on self' (ibid). Rice (1999) highlights the importance of speech and language therapists' views being 'based on ethical reasoning, not driven by emotion'.

Ethical conflict

Johns (1993) describes different types of conflicting values (a) within the client, (b) between the client and their family – interpersonal with other professionals, interpersonal with clients, intrapersonal – and (c) between the organisation and individual needs.

We suggest that such conflicts can be resolved through reflection and open discussion with colleagues by sharing experiences. Where the conflict involves the client and/or their family, discussion will take place with them.

LIVING WILLS AND ADVANCED DIRECTIVES (based on Foster, 1995)

Burgess (1994) states that 'knowing the patient's wishes in advance should also be taken into consideration when addressing the difficult question of whether or not to feed'. A living will is a document signed by a client and two independent witnesses (that is, not family members), which states that, under certain conditions, specific treatment or cessation of treatment should be adhered to (Foster, 1995). It is used in the event that a client becomes incapable of indicating or communicating their wishes later in their life, as with a client with progressing motor neurone disease (MND). These documents are most frequently made by people with terminal illness, but can be made by any competent adult at any stage of life. A number of charitable organisations have produced their own form of living will, for example the Terrence Higgins Trust in collaboration with The Centre of Medical Law and Ethics, Kings College, London. Foster provides an example of such indications given by a client with MND (*Nursing Times*, 1994): 'Where the application of life-sustaining procedures would serve only to artificially prolong the moment of my death, and where my physician determines that my death is imminent, whether or not life-sustaining procedures are utilised, I direct that such procedures are withheld or withdrawn, and that I am permitted to die naturally.'

The 'advanced directive' is often confused with a living will. It is in fact the generic term that includes living wills. Also included in an advanced directive are the following:

◆ *Surrogate consent.* This is where a person represents the client's interests in healthcare matters, and consents on behalf of the client once the client is no longer deemed competent to represent their own interests. Currently, no legal power is given to the next of kin or to those with enduring power of attorney in the United Kingdom.

◆ *Proxy consent.* This is the documentation of the individual's preference, even if it conflicts with what is seen to be in the client's best interest. It is also where a parent acts in respect of their child.

◆ *Treatment procedure.* This is the documentation in a client's medical records of the discussion and decisions regarding treatment, made prior to the end-stage of a terminal illness or in a period of remission. It is a record of the client's wishes for treatment at a later date, should the client not be deemed competent.

The legal status of living wills

The BMA (1999) states that advanced directives that are valid must be respected. A consultant physician who chooses to ignore a living will can be taken to court to ensure adherence to the client's wishes. At the time of writing the legal status of living wills has not been tested. Several reasons for this exist, including the following:

◆ The difficulty in establishing whether the individual substantially understands the full consequences of their actions, which may include the cessation of active medical intervention. The decision by the client must also be made following discussion with at least two doctors.

◆ Individuals change their minds. It is extremely difficult for clients to predict exactly how they will react when faced with the situation of making a decision in the end stages of an illness.

◆ The current circumstances must apply exactly to what was pre-directed in the will.

THE EFFECTS OF DEHYDRATION AND STARVATION ON THE CLIENT WHO IS DYING

There is an assumption that dehydration and starvation causes a painful death. However, on the basis of numerous case reports, data from hospice caregivers and empirical studies this is not the case (Slomka, 1995). Slomka reports that, when food and fluids are not desired by dying clients, administering them does not add to client comfort. Artificial nutrition and hydration in terminally ill clients may increase pain, oedema, respiratory congestion (and the need for suctioning), nausea and vomiting. Finally, she says that discomfort associated with dehydration resulting from thirst may be controlled with frequent mouth care, ice cubes and sips of fluids.

Dehydration has a sedative effect, which may increase a client's comfort, resulting in a painless and rapid death, within two to three days (Groher, 1990.)

ALTERNATIVE FEEDING AS A TREATMENT

Treatment is defined as:

◆ A clinical judgement made by the medical team
◆ Something which has to be consented to
◆ Something which can be refused
◆ Something which can be commenced or withdrawn (if not successful)

The primary goal of medical intervention is to benefit the client. Schneiderman *et al* (1990) argue that medical interventions that only sustain minimal function do not benefit the client overall. If a treatment fails, or ceases to provide an overall benefit to the client, it may be withdrawn or withheld. The focus of intervention then moves to controlling distressing symptoms and keeping the client comfortable (BMA, 1999). Fluid given via a tube is regarded as a medical treatment. The doctor is responsible for decisions to withhold, give or withdraw a medical treatment.

According to Lennard-Jones (1998), there is no distinction between withholding and withdrawing hydration and nutrition in ethical terms, but, from an emotive viewpoint, withdrawing may be more difficult.

Rice (1999) states that, 'depending on the underlying diagnosis and prognosis, the aim of care may be to either prolong life or to provide comfort during the terminal stages of dying ... A professional carer has a duty to prolong life but not to inappropriately prolong death'. BMA guidance suggests that the elements of basic care, such as oral nutrition using a cup or spoon and moistening of the mouth, should not be withdrawn, but that it should not be forced on a client 'who resists or refuses, or for whom the process of feeding becomes an unacceptable burden because of choking or inhalation of food or fluid'. In these cases, doctors should consider whether it would be of benefit to commence artificial feeding.

'In England, Wales and Northern Ireland, decisions to withdraw artificial nutrition and hydration from patients in Persistent Vegetative State (PVS) or conditions closely resembling PVS, currently require a Court declaration. The UK courts have not yet considered a case in relation to a patient with other irreversible conditions such as severe dementia or stroke' (BMA, 1999).

The importance of good communication in decision-making

Rice (1999) suggests there is an opportunity for speech and language therapists to facilitate clients' autonomy where they have communication impairments. The BMA guidance stresses the value of good communication between the doctor, client, relatives, carers and the multidisciplinary team. Sufficient time, resources and facilities need to be available for the team to make a thorough assessment of the client's best interests. Support and advice should be sought from other experienced colleagues when appropriate.

The BMA guidance goes on to say that, when a client is not able to communicate their wishes (for example, those with severe dementia, or those who have had a severe stroke, have little awareness of their surroundings and have no prospect of recovery), the doctors, in consultation with the relatives, carers and multidisciplinary team, have to decide whether providing life-prolonging treatment is in the client's best interests. There needs to be consensus among the team and relatives, and it will be reinforced that the client will continue to receive high-quality care. It suggests that any decision to withdraw artificial nutrition or hydration should be reviewed by a senior doctor outside the immediate team. This may be helpful and reassuring for both the families and the doctors.

GUIDELINES FOR GASTROSTOMY TUBE PLACEMENT (from Rabeneck *et al*, 1997)

Rabeneck *et al* (1997) ask what it is that the clinician seeks to achieve by suggesting a percutaneous endoscopic gastrostomy (PEG) tube. They say that the answer must be to benefit the client physiologically, that is, to provide improved nutritional status. The authors suggest that this be extended to improvements in the client's hydration status. Other positive changes in health outcomes are quality or length of life.

If recommending a PEG is likely to result in no improvements in nutritional or hydration status, then the team has no obligation to offer or perform the intervention. If the PEG is expected to improve the client's nutritional and hydration status but not their quality of life, as with, for example, a client in PVS, the doctor should recommend against having a PEG. If the PEG 'is expected to have a positive beneficial effect on all relevant clinical outcomes ... it should be recommended. However, when the intervention produces some favourable outcomes (eg prolonged life) and yet is also associated with unfavourable consequences (eg increased symptoms due to progressive underlying disease), then the overall clinical benefit is uncertain'. In this situation the authors recommend that the PEG be discussed with the client, but no recommendation made. 'Counselling should be completely informative but non-directive, allowing the patient to make the decision without the influence of the physician's recommendations.'

Rabeneck *et al* (1997) have devised a four-stage decision-making algorithm. First, does the client have an irreversible anorexia-cachectic syndrome, as seen in advanced cancer or AIDS? If so, PEG feeding will be of no nutritional benefit as the client will not be able to make use of the additional nutrients because of alterations in their metabolism. 'Unless the PEG tube is absolutely required for administration of medications, the procedure should not be offered.' Second, is the client in PVS? The minimal function of these clients means that it is not possible for them to experience any quality of life. A PEG tube may maintain their physiological function, but medical interventions that only sustain minimal function do not benefit the client overall (Schneiderman *et al*, 1990). The doctor should explain this to the client's family, offer a PEG tube and recommend against it. Third, does the client have a dysphagia without other deficits in their quality of life, as with, for example, clients with myasthenia gravis receiving drug therapy, whose only problem is dysphagia? They will gain full benefit from the nutrients delivered by the PEG tube, so one should be offered and recommended. Finally, does the client have dysphagia and deficits in quality of life? Examples include clients with reduced cognition, those with physical disabilities, or those with a progressive underlying disease (such as a bed-bound client with Alzheimer's disease). The doctor will identify the aspects of quality of life that are currently impaired and are likely to deteriorate as a result of disease progression. The doctor will explain the options of PEG tube placement and alternatives such as no PEG, as well as their positive and negative short- and long-term effects. These include discomfort during the procedure itself and complications such as infection at the stoma site, the tube becoming blocked and the potential for prolonging a life of decreased quality. Here it is for the client to decide, and not the doctor or clinician. Clients with the same impairments may view their quality of life very differently. According to the principle of autonomy, the doctor will non-directively discuss the PEG tube with the client. It will be presented as a trial of management that would be evaluated at intervals, particularly if adverse side effects on quality of life were experienced. An ethics committee will be consulted if the client is not able to participate in this discussion and they have no relatives or carers.

To conclude, Slomka (1995) suggests that, 'While any decision to forgo life-supporting treatment may cause anxiety and anguish for even the most experienced physician, the withholding or withdrawal of artificial nutrition and hydration appears to be the most difficult kind of decision to make and carry out', owing to the social and biological significance.

Chapter 13: Training Other Professionals

INTRODUCTION

In the preceding chapters the importance of working in collaboration with the multidisciplinary team in order to manage a client's dysphagia effectively has been emphasised. This chapter aims to raise awareness of some of the issues related to training other professional groups about swallowing impairment and management strategies in order to improve client care.

WHY PROVIDE TRAINING?

Training is an important component of the National Health Service's clinical governance strategy, which includes improving clinical effectiveness, facilitating lifelong learning and improving multidisciplinary working.

The pressures of increasing numbers of dysphagia referrals over the past decade have led many speech and language therapy services to introduce training programmes for members of the multidisciplinary team. Some of these programmes aim to reduce inappropriate referrals by training team members in the use of a screening procedure, for example for clients presenting with CVAs in Accident and Emergency departments. Information regarding a selection of these screening tools is provided at the end of this chapter. Also, packages have been developed to assist others in both the assessment and management of dysphagia (Badley & Tomlinson, 1995).

Benefits of training include the following

◆ Promotion of timely and appropriate referrals.
◆ Identification of clients with dysphagia who may not have been detected previously.
◆ Promotion of more appropriate management from the outset, which in turn promotes recovery and rehabilitation (RCSLT, 1996).
◆ Prevention of malnutrition and dehydration. This reduces the cost of alternative feeding and hydration, promotes wound healing and prevents the formation of pressure sores (Axelsson *et al*, 1988).
◆ Prevention of upper airway obstruction (may result in a costly admission to an intensive care bed).

- Prevention of chest infections, and in severe cases, death.

- Opportunities to improve understanding of the role of the speech and language therapist.

- Increased effectiveness in the multidisciplinary management of clients with dysphagia as a result of improved links and communication.

- Reduced client, family, carer and nurse anxiety regarding managing the client with dysphagia.

Training allows speech and language therapists 'to delegate tasks to other team members, the client or carer. The decision to delegate must be clinically motivated. Written and verbal instructions should be given, accompanied by demonstration and observation of the "proxy" therapist. Where a specified individual has been trained, they should be identified in the instructions. People acting under therapists' instructions must be given written information regarding the expected outcome of their actions, and what to do if difficulties arise. Speech and language therapists remain responsible for the "proxy" intervention if a task is delegated' (RCSLT, 1996).

Finally, training offers an opportunity to improve working relationships. Effective communication is essential within the team, and training provides a forum for discussion regarding roles and risk management issues while also offering continuing support. In-service training is increasingly attractive to other staff groups as a means of continuing their professional development, further improving the profile of dysphagia assessment and management.

TRAINING FORMATS

We suggest that training is most effective when the clinician has a working knowledge of the clients, their environment and their carers. Opportunities for teaching on a one-to-one basis are offered by every episode of client care (see Appendix IV for examples of advice sheets and dysphagia programmes). Group training sessions can then provide theory to support this practical work.

Dibben and James (1998) describe an 'intensive programme of instruction with subsequent one-to-one monitoring and supervision'. Training days are largely unsuccessful without follow-up: 'staff benefited from an opportunity to revisit or use that knowledge in a safe environment, hence the use of workbooks, which included practical scenarios bridging the gap between theory and practice'. In addition, the provision of a dysphagia resource pack (a minimum of one per ward) supports the group sessions. Turnover of staff means that it may be helpful to provide a rolling programme to maintain the benefits.

Wherever possible, it is advisable to involve those to be trained in setting up courses. For example, the clinician may devise the basic format, but involve nurse managers in agreeing the content and evaluation measures.

FURTHER ISSUES TO CONSIDER

Unidisciplinary or multidisciplinary trainers?

Is it appropriate for only the speech and language therapist to conduct the training, or will it be more effective to involve other professionals, particularly the dietitian, physiotherapist or specialist nurse (for example, one specialising in nutrition)? The decision will be influenced by the aims of the training sessions and other dysphagia-related projects running within a service, such as the introduction of nutritional assessment tools (see Chapter 9).

Who to train?

The clinician may wish to consider whether it is more beneficial to provide training to uniprofessional or multiprofessional groups, to a mix of staff on different grades, or to a mix of qualified and unqualified staff. Again, clarification of the purpose of the training sessions (see above) will assist the clinician in this decision.

The decision of whether to mix qualified nursing staff with healthcare assistants (HCAs) is worthy of further discussion. HCAs, although they are the most involved in feeding clients, and often the most experienced and aware of swallowing problems on a day-to-day basis, are not the decision-makers in clients' management. They may experience difficulties influencing the culture of a home or ward, and issues of empowerment may need to be addressed with nursing managers.

Domestic staff, volunteers, community staff and families are often overlooked when training courses are being set up, yet they are equally in need of training. The Scottish Intercollegiate Guidelines Network (1997) advises that catering staff require 'information and training to enable them to appreciate the importance of specific food consistencies and to prepare appropriate meals or food items, with any necessary nutritional supplementation advised by a dietitian'. The potential risks of aspiration at night time – when there are lower levels of qualified staff on duty and difficulties seating clients – suggest that training for night staff is important, despite the challenges presented to this group of attending sessions.

Education in dysphagia is often part of the professional training courses of nurses and doctors. Increasingly the UK National Vocational Qualifications (NVQs) curriculum includes sessions relating to swallowing disorders and nutrition.

Schemes to train 'proxy' therapists

Dysphagia 'link nurses' are an increasing feature of the assessment and management of swallowing difficulties (Badley & Tomlinson, 1995; Dibben & James, 1998; Giles & Davison, 1996; Jones, 1998; O'Loughlin & Shanley, 1998; Riches, 1991). Their roles, levels of responsibility, title, training and supervision vary from unit to unit. Training resources have been developed from these projects (Heritage & Knapp, 1992; O'Loughlin & Shanley, 1996; Badley & Tomlinson, 1995).

Badley and Tomlinson (1995) identified issues for speech and language therapists supervising professional groups who work to different standards and with different skills: 'Nurses bring to their new role well-developed skills of applying their observations to the broader medical context [but] nurse training is far more procedurally based. Therefore a large part of the training programme has involved developing detailed observational skills of the swallowing process whilst providing a clear-cut procedure with precise referral criteria.'

Evaluating the effectiveness of training

Since training is often introduced to reduce the number of inappropriate referrals and to aid referring agents in prioritising and managing clients more effectively, referral patterns may be studied to determine the effectiveness of training. Referrals may remain high if the training equips assessors to identify subtle or mild swallowing problems.

Pre- and post-training questionnaires may be utilised to determine the level of acquired knowledge and the application of that knowledge. Written feedback relating to the staff's levels of confidence (for example, when assessing whether aspiration is present, or observing for signs of aspiration) prior to and following the sessions are to be used with caution – confidence may decrease initially as staff understand more fully the implications of an impaired swallow. Course participants can be encouraged to return post-training questionnaires if they are provided with a certificate of attendance on receipt of the questionnaire.

Further methods of evaluation include (a) outcome measures, for example incidence of chest infections, length of time non-oral feeding routes are required; (b) qualitative observations (adherence to guidelines, use of recommended utensils and crockery); (c) care plan audits; (d) monitoring complaints, and (e) feedback from peer review sessions and support meetings.

SCREENING TOOLS FOR OTHER PROFESSIONAL GROUPS

A number of screening tools for a range of other professionals have been developed to aid prompt and appropriate referral to the dysphagia team, and to aid the management of a client in the interim between referral and assessment: for example, the screening of an acutely ill patient admitted to hospital over the weekend when speech and language therapy cover is not available. Effective use of screening tools may be achieved if supported by a staff-training programme that includes information on the basic anatomy and physiology of swallowing, and signs and symptoms of dysphagia. A selection of tools in use in the United Kingdom is detailed below.

Scottish Intercollegiate Guidelines Network, pilot edition (1997)

These guidelines are for use by a trained nurse or doctor to screen clients who have sustained a CVA. The client is required to swallow a set amount of water. The practitioner is directed to signs which would indicate an appropriate referral to the speech and language therapy service for full assessment.

The swallow test (Crockford and Smithard, 1997)

This swallow test further developed the work of DePippo *et al* (see below), resulting in a two-minute screening test for use by doctors and nurses that would be specific, sensitive, and require a minimum of training and minimal readily available equipment. Early results indicate an improvement in detection of dysphagia, although further research is under way to develop the test. It is in use in a number of acute hospital units in the United Kingdom.

A timed test (Nathadwarawala et al, 1994)

This has the potential to offer an early diagnosis of swallowing problems for those clients attending neurology outpatient clinics who may, or may not, complain of dysphagia. The client is timed drinking 150ml of water as fast as possible, but safely, and instructed to stop if they experience any discomfort. The number of swallows is also counted by observing movements of the thyroid cartilage. From these observations the swallowing speed and average volume per swallow are calculated. Reduced speed of swallowing is viewed as a compensatory strategy that may be utilised in chronic neurological diseases before overt clinical signs develop.

The Burke dysphagia screening test (DePippo et al, 1994)

This aims to identify the relative risk of pneumonia, recurrent upper airway obstruction and death. If identified as high-risk, the client is referred for videofluoroscopy and then a treatment programme is devised. This can be used by any trained healthcare professional, who will then refer the client on to the speech and language therapist for further assessment and management.

The swallowing checklist (Rainbow, 1998, unpublished)

This quick-to-administer checklist is provided to support training sessions to a range of professional groups, particularly student doctors and qualified nursing staff, and to aid appropriate referral to the speech and language therapy team.

Acute signs

1 Does the person's medical condition alert you to possible dysphagia (for example, CVA, head and neck cancer, progressive neurological condition, learning difficulty)?

2 Does the person cough or choke when eating or drinking?

3 Does the person have (a) a cough reflex, (b) a swallow reflex?

4 Does the person have reduced lip, jaw or tongue movement?

5 Does the person have good oral hygiene? Does residue of food or drink collect in his/her mouth?

6 Can the person maintain a square sitting position?

7 Can the person cope with his/her saliva?

8 Does the person's voice sound 'gurgly'?

9 Can the person swallow (a) liquids, (b) semi-solids, (c) solids?

10 Does the person experience severe discomfort or pain on swallowing?

11 Is the person easily distracted so that he/she cannot give their full attention to safe swallowing?

12 Does the person tire quickly when eating or drinking?

13 Does the person show signs of aspiration, particularly (a) a chest infection affecting the right lung base, (b) a spiking temperature (indicating acute infection)?

14 Can the person self-feed?

Chronic signs

1 Weight loss

2 Chronic or recurrent repetitive chest infections

3 Lack of interest in food/refusal to eat

4 Poor hydration and/or nutrition

When you have identified these signs

Can you reduce any of the risk factors? Should you refer to the speech and language therapist and/or dietitian for a fuller assessment?

Working with people who have dysphagia is a very rewarding experience. Providing the client, their relatives, carers and the multidisciplinary team with information and training can demystify dysphagia, enhance the quality of the swallowing management, improve outcomes and foster a philosophy of enabling and independence.

Appendixes

Appendix I

EASY-TO-SWALLOW FOODS

These can be fortified if necessary.

Root vegetables	Diced or mashed turnips, swede, young parsnips, carrots, sweet potatoes
Other vegetables	Cauliflower (including cauliflower cheese), broccoli (soft), courgettes, avocado
Potatoes	Boiled, baked, mashed (with butter)
Meat	Pâté, mince, very finely chopped meats in gravy
Fish	Baked/grilled with sauce, plaice/sole/skate, pilchards/ sardines, eg, in tomato sauce, boil-in-the-bag fish in sauces, fish with a fine texture rather than flaky coarse texture (haddock/cod/coley tend to be too solid)
Eggs	Omelette, scrambled or poached. Need to cook thoroughly because of risk of salmonella
Tinned	Baked beans, spaghetti, macaroni cheese, ravioli, cream of soups
Fruit	Bananas, stewed apples, apple purée, ripe peaches, ripe pears, papaya
Other puddings	Ice-cream, sorbets, mousse, blancmange, jelly, rice pudding, tapioca, yogurt (not liked by all older people), custard (including egg custard), soya puddings
Dairy	Cottage cheese
Cereals	Weetabix (plenty of milk), porridge

Marks *et al* (2001) suggest the following 'Classification of Food Textures with Food Examples':

TEXTURE CLASSIFICATION	EXAMPLE OF FOOD
hard	apple
chewy	cooked meat
soft	cake, bread/butter (no crust)
liquid hard lump	muesli
liquid soft lump	cornflakes and milk
thickened soft lump	plain yogurt and banana
thickened hard lump	stew with chewy meat
liquid	milk, water and orange juice
slide down easily	butter, peanut butter, mousse

a soft diet, for example using minced meat, flaked fish, soft fruit, vegetables and mashed potato (with food enrichment: butter/margarine, milk powder)

a soft smooth diet where food is soft and mashed, for example puréed meat with gravy, fish in sauce, mashed soft vegetables, soft mashed potatoes, milk pudding, fruit yogurts (with food enrichment)

a purée diet (homogenised), where food is puréed using a blender and additional fluid is added: for example puréed meat, potato, vegetables and fruit, smooth yogurt, mousse, ground rice pudding

Appendix II

SUPPLIERS OF EQUIPMENT

Drooling swallow reminder brooch, available from Bath Institute of Medical Engineering, the Wolfson Centre, RUH, Combe Park, Bath, BA1 3NG

Kapitex Healthcare Ltd, Kapitex House, 1 Sandbeck Way, Wetherby, West Yorkshire, LS22 7GH (for 'flexicups' and 'dysphagia cups')

Pat Saunders valved drinking straw available from Nottingham Rehab Supplies, 17 Ludlow Hill Road, Melton Road, West Bridgford, Nottingham, NG2 6HD

Phagia Viscometer meddiet@med-diet.com

Plak-Vac trademark@worldnet.att.net

Appendix III

WEBSITES

American Speech and Hearing Association www.asha.org

Aspiration – a slide that can be viewed
www.kumc.edu/instruction/medicine/pathology/ed/ch_12/c12_s12.html

British Healthcare Internet Association www.bhia.org/

British Medical Association www.bma.org.uk

Carbonated drinks reference www.dysphagia-diet.com/newsl.html

Changing Faces – support organisation for people with facial disfigurements
www.changingfaces.co.uk

Chartered Society of Physiotherapy www.csp.org.uk

Cochrane Library on effectiveness of healthcare www.cochrane.co.uk

College of Occupational Therapy www.cot.uk

Department of Health www.doh.gov.uk

Dysphagia Diet Website www.dysphagia-diet.com/index.html

Dysphagia Journal www.link.springer-ny.com

Dysphagia Resource Centre, by Phyllis Palmer www.dysphagia.com/

Headway – the national association for people with head injuries
www.headway.org.uk

Healthgate: a company publishing medical information on the net
www.healthgate.com/

Institute of Neurotoxicology and Neurological Disorders:
ALS materials: www.innd.org/als.html
Alzheimer's www.innd.org/alzheim.html
Parkinson's www.innd.org/parkinsn.html

Jeri Logemann www.nuinfo.nwu.edu/csd/FACULTY/logemann.html

Katherine Yorkston www.ticeinfo.com

Medline www.nlm.him.gov/

Michael Groher www.menudirect.com/consistencymod/infocenter_drgroher.html

National Centre for Clinical Excellence www.Nice.org.uk

National Library of Medicine's MEDLINE www.medscape.com

Neurology Web-Forum
www.demOnmac.mgh.harvard.edu:80/neurowebforum/neurowebforum.html

Passy–Muir Speaking Valves info@passy-muir.com

Pneumonia information
www.meddean.luc.edu/lumen/MedEd/medicine/pulmonar/pul4.html

Royal College of Nursing www.rcn.org.uk

Royal College of Physicians www.rcplondon.ac.uk

Royal College of Speech and Language Therapists www.rcslt.org

Scottish Intercollegiate Guidelines Network www.sign.ac.uk

Speech Pathology Australia www.vicnet.net.au/~sppathau

Speechmark Publishing – useful links and resources for speech and language
therapists including dysphagia www.speechmark.net

Support organisation for people with lymphomas www.lymphoma.org.uk

The Kings Fund www.kingsfund.org.uk

The Lupus Trust – St Thomas' Hospital, London, UK www.infotech.demon.co.uk

The Stroke Association www.stroke.org.uk

The Whole Brain Atlas www.med.harvard.edu/AANLIB/home/html

Traumatic Brain Injury – Perspectives Network Homepage www.tbi.org

UK Resuscitation Council Enquiries@resus.org.uk

Mailing lists

Dysphagia subscribe dysphagia@cyberport.com to majordomo@cyberport.com

or Majordomo@medline.com

Appendix IV

EXAMPLES OF WRITTEN GUIDELINES, MONITORING FORMS AND RATING SCALES

SUGGESTIONS FOR PREPARING GUIDELINES

◆ Describe the swallowing problem

◆ Describe the philosophy of approach (if appropriate)

◆ Make the aim explicit

◆ Describe the expected outcome if possible

◆ Present information in a clear, jargon-free and logical format

◆ Agree the guidelines with the client and carers

◆ Provide a monitoring form

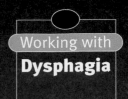

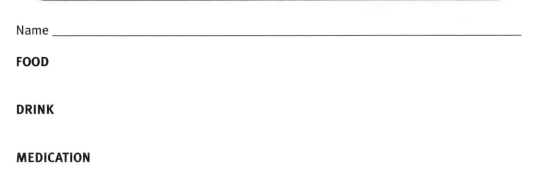

EXAMPLE 1: SPEECH & LANGUAGE THERAPY
EATING & DRINKING GUIDELINES

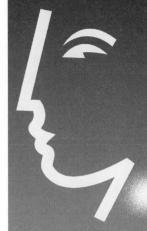

Name _____

FOOD

DRINK

MEDICATION

EAT/DRINK ONLY WHEN

◆ Fully alert (reduce distractions if necessary)

◆ In upright sitting position, preferably in a chair

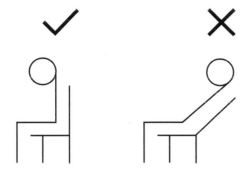

• Sitting upright
• Head forward

STOP IF

◆ Coughing/choking (up to 2 minutes after food/drink)

◆ Voice becomes 'gurgly'

◆ Showing signs of fatigue, eg swallowing getting slower

SPECIFIC INFORMATION

AFTER EATING/DRINKING

◆ Remain upright for 20/30 minutes

◆ Check mouth is clear and clean/mouth care

Contact your nurse/speech and language therapist if you notice any difficulties with eating or drinking

Speech and language therapist _____

Bleep _____ Date _____

Photocopiable

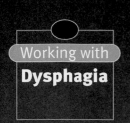

EXAMPLE 2: THERAPY PROGRAMME TO HELP DROOLING

INTRODUCTION

Dampness in the corners of the mouth and drooling can be very embarrassing. People who have a problem with drooling tend to swallow their saliva less frequently than those who do not. Drooling is often worse in the afternoon or evening, as people become more tired and it is harder to make the swallow start promptly.

WHAT IS THE PURPOSE OF SPEECH AND LANGUAGE THERAPY FOR DROOLING?

The aim is to increase your awareness of swallowing saliva to give you more control over your drooling.

The main goal of therapy is to **CONSCIOUSLY SWALLOW MORE OFTEN** so that the saliva does not build up inside your mouth and then cause the drooling.

WHAT DOES THE THERAPY INVOLVE AT HOME?

1 **Drooling Awareness Charts**

Please fill in the attached sheets for 7 days (see Figure A.3):

- once in the **morning** for 5 minutes
- once in the **afternoon** for 5 minutes
- once in the **evening** for 5 minutes

1 Choose times when you can sit in a chair, hold the sheet of paper and a pen.

2 Use the kitchen timer supplied, turn it on for 5 minutes.

3 **Mark on the form every time that you notice you have swallowed your saliva.**

4 When the timer rings, put down the pen and paper and stop.

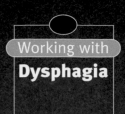

EXAMPLE 2: THERAPY PROGRAMME TO HELP DROOLING

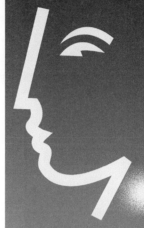

2   Swallow Reminder Brooch

Use this every day for 4 weeks.

1   Switch on the brooch by pressing the little white button on the back.

2   A small 'beep' will be heard (if not, the battery may be flat).

3   Either pin the brooch to your shirt, blouse, jacket or jumper, **or** put it round your neck using the chain supplied.

4   Use the kitchen timer again, turning it on for 30 minutes this time.

5   Every time you hear the 'beep' please **consciously swallow your saliva.**

6   When the timer rings, take the brooch off.

7   Press the white button again to turn it off.

Photocopiable

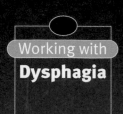

Working with Dysphagia

EXAMPLE 3: DROOLING RATING SCALE

Name _____

Date _____

Rated by Client ☐ or Carer ☐ (please tick)

	Excessive dryness of mouth	No excess saliva	Excess of saliva in mouth without drooling	Mild to moderate drooling: needs occasional wiping	Continuous drooling: wet clothes or constant use of handkerchief or tissue
Sitting					
Standing or walking					
In bed					
Talking					
Eating/drinking					
Concentrating on activity, eg dressing					

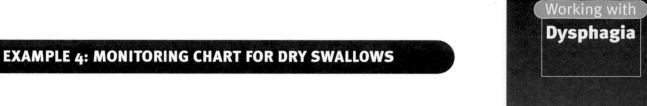

EXAMPLE 4: MONITORING CHART FOR DRY SWALLOWS

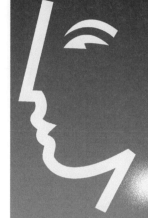

Name

Please select 5 minutes, 3 times a day and put a tick in the appropriate box each time you swallow.

Day	1	2	3	4	5	6	7
Morning							
Afternoon							
Evening							

Photocopiable

© L Marks & D Rainbow, 2001

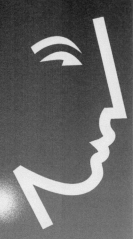

EXAMPLE 5: DESENSITISATION PROGRAMME FOR JANE S

PROBLEM

Jane is hypersensitive around and in her mouth. This means that she may make movements such as pursing her lips, abnormal grimacing, chewing and yawning, or actually trigger a bite reflex. Hypersensitivity may occur when her face or mouth is touched, particularly when offering her a spoonful of food, her cup or toothbrush. This can make it hard for her to open her mouth and therefore difficult for the carer to give her food or drink and to brush her teeth afterwards. It is important for mouth care to be done to maintain good oral hygiene, to prevent build up of plaque and bacteria, which could be at risk of going the wrong way, into her lungs.

AIM

To reduce oral hypersensitivity using touch to help eating, drinking and mouth care.

BEFORE YOU START

◆ Reduce any background noise and distractions (turn off any music or the TV).

◆ Tell her what you are going to do at each stage and count her in, so that she can anticipate what is going to happen and when. For example 'I'm going to touch your arm – 1, 2, 3' (and then touch).

◆ This should take a maximum of 5 minutes, and be done every time before she is offered food or drink, or before she is moved or washed.

PROGRAMME

1 Start working with gentle but firm touch, starting at the area furthest from her face and work up her body to her face (hands, lower arms, upper arms, shoulders, back of neck, back of head, crown and so on). If she starts showing even the smallest signs of increased tone or reflexes mentioned above, go back and work more on the part which started this response.

2 Move up the back of her neck and head, coming gradually over the top of the skull, towards the forehead, then to the cheeks and down towards the mouth. Again, the actions should be carried out with gentle, but firm stroking

Photocopiable

© L Marks & D Rainbow, 2001

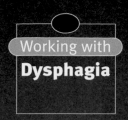

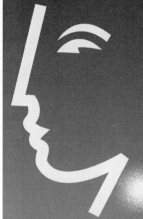

EXAMPLE 5: DESENSITISATION PROGRAMME FOR JANE S

movements. It is quite common to find that the lower half of the face, around the mouth and inside the oral cavity is more sensitive than the top half of the face.

3   Using a gloved finger, stroke firmly three times above the top lip from right to left. There may be grimacing, chewing or yawning at this point. If there is, see if it helps to repeat until it reduces. Repeat by stroking below the bottom lip.

4   Next, stroke the top lip itself several times. Repeat on the bottom lip itself also.

5   Now moisten your gloved finger with water. Slide this into Jane's mouth and run the pad of your finger along her top right gum from front to back, in a slow rhythmical way. On the third time, turn the finger so that the pad touches the cheek, then stretch the cheek out and then remove the finger. Then do this on the left side. Repeat this on the lower gum. This will often reduce tension and relax the tongue, bringing it more forward in the mouth.

6   Now it should be easier to give Jane teaspoons of food and very thick fluids, and to perform mouth care.

Jane will benefit from this programme only if it can be performed several times a day (ideally a minimum of three times a day).

It may take some time before her hypersensitivity reduces, so please keep going. She will be reviewed in three days' time. Many thanks for your help.

Signed _____ Speech & Language Therapist

Date _____

Photocopiable

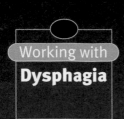

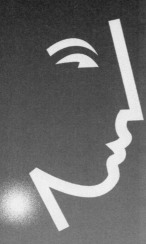

EXAMPLE 6: AN ORAL HYGIENE PROGRAMME

CURRENT DIFFICULTIES

Doug has difficulty swallowing, owing to reduced movement of his tongue. Sometimes the swallow is very sluggish and sometimes he is unable to swallow. His cough is very weak. These factors make him at risk of aspiration, that is, food or drink going into the lungs.

AIM OF THIS PROGRAMME

◆ To maintain good oral hygiene

◆ To keep Doug's mouth feeling comfortable

◆ To reduce the risk of infections in his mouth

ORAL HYGIENE PROGRAMME

◆ Needs to be carried out five or six times a day.

◆ Doug needs supervision but can carry out the mouth care himself.

◆ Use pink foam swabs and water. Soak the swab and then gently squeeze out any excess; the swab should remain damp.

◆ Give Doug the swab and tell him which part of his mouth to clean. Only move on to the next area when the previous one is clean.

◆ Areas to clean:
   - tongue, including sides and back
   - between teeth and cheeks, both upper and lower teeth
   - roof of his mouth including the back

◆ It is important to do the programme after brushing his teeth, as some toothpaste tends to sit on the back of his tongue and the roof of his mouth. Doug is not aware that it is there and his swallow is not strong enough to clear it away.

◆ Each session is likely to take a minimum of 5 minutes.

Photocopiable

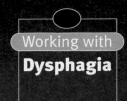
EXAMPLE 7: WAYS TO HELP COPE WITH SALIVA

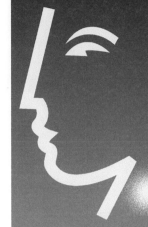

John drools as he has difficulty swallowing his saliva. He can usually swallow normally, but will only do this when he has food or drink in his mouth. The amount of saliva in his mouth is too small for him to notice in order to swallow. Sitting forward makes the difficulty worse.

Here are some suggestions to help. They rely on others, rather than John himself, to make changes.

MEDICATION TO DRY UP THE SALIVA

This has to be prescribed by the doctor who will advise on the correct dose and possible side effects. Options include hyoscine patches or Kwells.

GOOD MOUTH CARE

John's saliva is very thick, as he has reduced oral hygiene. Try to encourage him to clean his mouth, by using a mouthwash, swilling with water, or using foam swabs (but be careful with these in case he accidentally bites off the foam).

DRINKS

Some drinks are more likely than others to make someone produce saliva. Water is best because it is cleansing. Alcohol and tobacco have a drying effect on the mouth.

TISSUES AND PROMPTS TO USE THEM

It is helpful to give John tissues and remind him to wipe his mouth as often as possible.

Photocopiable

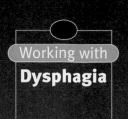

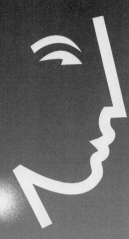

EXAMPLE 8: EXAMPLE OF THE TRANSITION FROM LONG-TERM, NON-ORAL FEEDING TO TASTES FOR PLEASURE

These swallowing guidelines are designed to provide Alice with pleasurable opportunities to eat, preferably at lunchtime in the dining area with other residents. It is suggested that only a few nurses (three, say) give Alice food.

BEFORE YOU START

Alice will be sitting upright in a chair

Make sure that you are sitting down next to her

FOODS TO USE

Desserts: custard, chocolate sauce, crème caramel, ice-cream, jelly, mousse, sago, rice pudding, yogurts, fromage frais

Offer small quantities only: 10 spoonfuls maximum

GUIDELINES

1 Half fill a flat dessertspoon

2 With your hand on Alice's, help her feed herself

3 Alice takes the dessert from the spoon with her tongue and lips

4 Feel for the swallow (see Figure 1.7, page 11)

5 Praise her when you feel the swallow

6 Encourage at least one more swallow to ensure that it is all cleared away

7 After a pause of at least 3 minutes, you can offer Alice the next spoonful

Stop if Alice's breathing deteriorates, for example becoming wheezy, or if Alice becomes tired.

Please record all results (including any coughing) in the nursing folder.

Photocopiable

© L Marks & D Rainbow, 2001

230

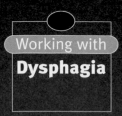

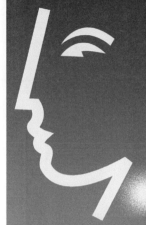

EXAMPLE 9: POST-ACUTE DYSPHAGIA

Dan may forget to swallow his food, and may keep on chewing it. Please follow the advice below carefully to avoid this and reduce the risk of aspiration.

◆ Dan needs to be supervised for all food and drink.

◆ He needs to be sitting up in his chair for all food, drink and medication.

◆ He needs to be wearing his false teeth for all food and drink.

◆ He needs to feed himself: give him the cup/glass, slice of bread and so on. He has difficulty seeing his food, so you may need to fill the spoon/fork for him, but then give it to him to put in his mouth.

◆ If he has been chewing for a long time, remind him to stop chewing and swallow. He may need reminding twice per mouthful.

◆ Try to avoid purée. He can manage a normal diet.

◆ If you have any queries or concerns, please contact the Speech and Language Therapy Department.

Photocopiable

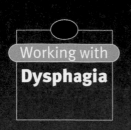

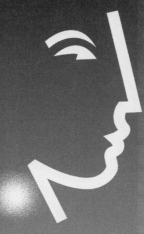

EXAMPLE 10: CHRONIC DYSPHAGIA

There is a risk that Phil may choke, or that food/drink may go into his lungs unless everyone feeding him adheres to the guidelines below.

AGITATION

Phil can be very agitated at times – he calls out, or pushes himself back in his chair. Try to identify times when Phil is quieter and make sure that he is as calm as possible before you give him food or drink. He may need to be reminded to sit down, and to swallow.

REDUCED ALERTNESS

At other times Phil may be less alert than is ideal for eating and drinking. If he appears particularly tired or 'switched off', **do not feed him**. Wait until he is more alert. If he continues to be drowsy, it may be necessary to give him nutrition and hydration via his gastrostomy on that day.

DRINKS

All drinks need to be thickened to a milk shake consistency. It takes about EIGHT minutes to give Phil half a glass of fluid, so be sure that you have sufficient time before starting.

Use a soupspoon to give Phil fluids. Show him the half-full spoon for a second. He can then respond by opening his mouth. Place the spoon on the centre of his tongue so that he can take the drink off it. Never pour the fluid into his mouth.

Pause for at least 30 seconds between mouthfuls.

Photocopiable

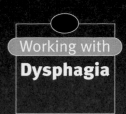

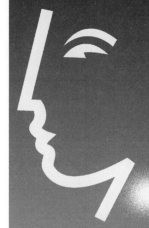

EXAMPLE 10: CHRONIC DYSPHAGIA

FOODS

Phil does not chew and is often slow to swallow a mouthful. He needs softer foods with plenty of gravy, sauce, custard, cream, butter, and so on to moisten them.

A fork is ideal for giving him main courses. Use a soupspoon for desserts, but try not to overfill it. Make sure that he has a moment to see what is on the fork/spoon before putting it in his mouth. This way he will be better prepared for it. As with the fluids, place the fork/spoon on the centre of his tongue so that he can take the food off it.

Pause for at least 30 seconds between mouthfuls.

POSSIBLE PROBLEMS

◆ Phil is very agitated. If you cannot identify why Phil is so agitated, and it is not possible to calm him down, it may be more appropriate not to give him food or a drink at that time.

◆ Phil coughs. This may be because Phil is too agitated, you are not pausing for long enough between mouthfuls, or he has forgotten to swallow. It may be necessary to stop, or remind him to swallow.

Photocopiable

© L Marks & D Rainbow, 2001

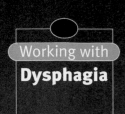

Working with
Dysphagia

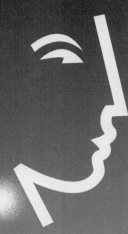

EXAMPLE 11: WARNING SIGNS TO INITIATE RE-REFERRAL
(for example, for a client with a progressive neurological disease)

AREAS OF SWALLOWING TO MONITOR

IF ANY OF THE THINGS BELOW START TO HAPPEN, CONTACT THE SPEECH AND LANGUAGE THERAPIST

◆ Coughing on food or drink increases

◆ Regular chest infections

◆ Chewing becomes difficult

◆ Client or the carers are worried

◆ Client's voice sounds 'gurgly', particularly after food or drink

Photocopiable

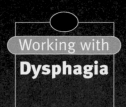

EXAMPLE 12: A THERMAL STIMULATION MONITORING FORM

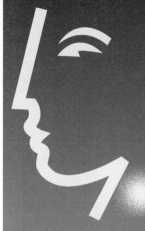

Date and time	Outcome, eg swallow triggered? If yes, amount of delay	Any problems/ observations, eg too tired to participate, gagging?	Nurse/ Therapist Initials

Photocopiable

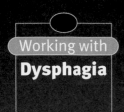

EXAMPLE 13: AN ORAL INTAKE/SWALLOWING MONITORING FORM

Date and time	Food/drink taken triggered? If yes, amount of delay	Outcome, eg required prompts, coughing, declined	Nurse/ Therapist Initials

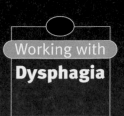

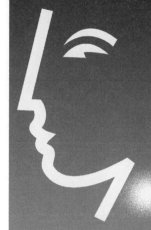

EXAMPLE 14: SMALL STEP PROGRESSION FOR TEACHING A SUPRAGLOTTIC SWALLOW

STAGE 1

Breathe in through your mouth

Hold it, keeping your mouth closed

Let out the air of your mouth with a cough

STAGE 2

Breathe in through your mouth

Hold it, keeping your mouth closed

Continue to hold your breath while opening and closing your mouth

Let out the air with a cough

STAGE 3

Breathe in through your mouth

Hold it

Continue to hold your breath while opening your mouth, and mime putting in
a spoon

Close your mouth

Swallow

Let out the air with a cough

STAGE 4

Breathe in through your mouth

Hold it

Continue to hold your breath while opening your mouth, and mime putting in
a spoon

Close your mouth

Swallow

Swallow again

Let out the air with a cough

STAGE 5

Breathe in through your mouth

Hold it

Open your mouth and put in a spoonful of food/drink

Close your mouth

Swallow

Swallow again

Let out the air with a cough

Photocopiable

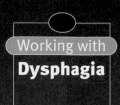

Working with
Dysphagia

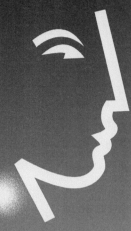

EXAMPLE 15: BLUE DYE TEST FOR ASPIRATION FOR CLIENTS WITH TRACHEOSTOMIES

◆ Dilute blue food colouring or methylene blue with sterile water

◆ Suction and deflate the cuff, or partially deflate the cuff

◆ Place two to three drops on the client's tongue with a syringe

◆ Ask the client to swallow their saliva

◆ Note any voice change and encourage the client to cough or throat clear as needed

◆ Ask the client to take a sip of blue water

◆ Note any voice change and encourage the client to cough or throat clear as needed

◆ Suction

◆ Allow the client to rest if required, and partially reinflate the cuff if necessary

◆ Resuction

◆ If no traces of blue are noted, continue with larger amounts, or other consistencies. If traces are found, terminate the test and consider trying different consistencies

◆ Reinflate the cuff as required

◆ Ask the nursing and physiotherapy staff to monitor the stoma site during the day, where the tracheostomy meets the skin of the neck, and to document the presence or absence of traces of blue dye

Photocopiable

Bibliography

American Speech–Language–Hearing Association, 1999a, 'Instrumental Diagnostic Procedures for Swallowing', *Position Statement III*, pp27–38.

American Speech–Language–Hearing Association, 1999b, 'Knowledge and skills needed by Speech–Language Pathologists Providing Services to Patients/Clients', *Guidelines III*, pp113–19.

Appleton J & Machin J, 1995, *Working with Oral Cancer*, Speechmark/Winslow Press, Bicester.

Avery-Smith W, Rosen A & Dellarosa D, 1997, *Dysphagia Evaluation Protocol*, Therapy Skill Builders, ISBN 1-800-228-0752.

Axelsson K, Asplund K, Norberg A & Alafuzoff I, 1988, 'Nutritional Status in Patients with Acute Stroke', *Acta Med Scand* 224, pp217–24.

Badley K & Tomlinson P, 1995, 'Are we prepared to share the management of dysphagia with nurses and are they prepared to take it on?', *RCSLT Bulletin* June, pp8–9.

Barofsky I & Fontaine KR, 1998, 'Do Psychogenic Patients Have an Eating Disorder?', *Dysphagia* 13, pp24–7.

Barton S & McLaughlin S, 1997, 'Enjoy your Meal', *Speech and Language Therapy in Practice* Summer, pp4–5.

Bell S, 1996, 'Use of Passy-Muir Tracheostomy Speaking Valve in Mechanically Ventilated Neurological Patients', *Critical Care Nurse* 16 (1), pp63–8.

Bleach N, 1993, 'The Gag Reflex and Aspiration: a retrospective analysis of 120 patients assessed by videofluoroscopy', *Clinical Otolaryngology* 18, pp303–7.

Blitzer A, 1990, 'Approaches to the Patient with Aspiration and Swallowing Disabilities', *Dysphagia* 5, pp129–37.

Boolkin L, 1998, 'The Management of Dysphagia in Tracheostomy and Ventilator-Dependent Head-injured Patients', *Australian Communication Quarterly*, Winter, pp6–8.

Brin MF & Younger D, 1988, 'Neurologic Disorders and Aspiration', *Otolaryngologic Clinics of North America* 21 (4), pp691–9.

British Medical Association, 1997, *BMA New Guide to Medicines and Drugs*, Dorling Kindersley, London.

British Medical Association, 1999, BMA publishes new ethical guidance on withdrawal of treatment, BMA press release 23 June, London.

Brown BP & Sonies BC, 1997, 'Diagnostic Methods to Evaluate Swallowing Other Than Barium Contrast', Perlman AL and Schulze-Delrieu K (eds), *Deglutition and its Disorders: Anatomy, Physiology, Clinical Diagnosis, and Management*, Singular Publishing , San Diego.

Burgess A, 1994, 'Dilemmas of deglutition', *CSLT Bulletin* August, pp4–5.

Camden and Islington Community Health Services NHS Trust, 1999, 'Food Hygiene Policy'.

Cherney L, Canterieri C & Pannell J, 1986, *Chicago Clinical Evaluation of Dysphagia*, Aspen Publishers, USA.

Cichero J, 1996, 'Cervical Auscultation – An Assessment of the Sounds of Swallowing', *Australian Communication Quarterly* Spring, pp22–4.

Chi-Fishman G & Sonies B, 1998, 'New Insights into Motor Strategy and Control in Sequential Swallowing', abstract of scientific paper presented at the 7th Annual Dysphagia Research Society Meeting, New Orleans, Louisiana.

Crary MA, 1995, 'A Direct Intervention Program for Chronic Neurogenic Dysphagia Secondary to Brainstem Stroke', *Dysphagia* 10, pp6–8.

Crary M, Glowasky A & Antonelli P, 1995, 'Transcutaneous Injection of Botulinum Toxin A to Facilitate Opening of the Pharyngooesophageal Segment', abstract from the 4th Annual Dysphagia Research Society Meeting, USA.

Crockford C & Smithard D, 1997, 'The Swallow Test', *RCSLT Bulletin* January, pp7–8.

Davies AE, Kidd D, Stone SP & MacMahon J, 1995, 'Pharyngeal sensation and gag reflex in healthy subjects', *The Lancet* 345, pp487–8.

De Paso W, 1991, 'Aspiration Pneumonia', *Clinics in Chest Medicine* 12 (2).

DePippo KL, Holas MA & Reding MJ, 1994, 'The Burke dysphagia screening test; validation for its use in patients with stroke', *Arch Phys Med Rehabil* 75, pp1284–6.

DeVault K, 1997, 'Incomplete Upper Oesophageal Sphincter Relaxation: Association with Achalasia but Not Other Oesophageal Motility Disorders', *Dysphagia* 12, pp157–60.

Dibben S & James J, 1998, 'Dysphagia Training for Qualified Nursing Staff', Speech and Language Therapy Service, Central Nottinghamshire Healthcare (NHS) Trust, unpublished.

Dikeman KJ & Kazandjian MS, 1995, *Communication and Swallowing Management of Tracheostomized and Ventilator-Dependent Adults,* Singular Publishing Group, San Diego.

Di Vito J, 1998, 'Cervical Osteophytic Dysphagia: Single and Combined Mechanisms', *Dysphagia* 13, pp58–61.

Dodds W, 1989, 'The Physiology of Swallowing', *Dysphagia* 3, pp171–8.

Drug and Therapeutics Bulletin, 1996, 'Malnourished Inpatients: Overlooked and Undertreated', *Drug and Therapeutics* Bulletin 34 (8).

Duvoisin, RC, 1982, *Parkinson's Disease: A Guide for Patient and Family,* New York, Raven Press

Dworkin J & Nadal J, 1991, 'Non Surgical Treatment of Drooling in a Patient with Closed Head Injury and Severe Dysarthria', *Dysphagia* 6, pp40–9.

Evans Morris S & Dunn Klein M, 1987, *Pre-Feeding Skills – A Comprehensive Resource for Feeding Development,* Therapy Skill Builders, Tucson, Arizona.

Feinberg M, Knebl J & Tully J, 1996, 'Prandial Aspiration and Pneumonia in an Elderly Population Followed over 3 Years', *Dysphagia* 11, pp104–9.

Foster C, 1995, 'Living Wills with specific reference to Motor Neurone Disease and Alternative Feeding', *unpublished*.

Finucane TE & Bynum JPW, 1996, 'Use of tube feeding to prevent aspiration pneumonia', *The Lancet* 348, pp1421–4.

Fonda D, Schwarz J & Clinnick S, 1995, 'Parkinsonian Medication One Hour Before Meals Improves Symptomatic Swallowing: A Case Study', *Dysphagia* 10, pp165–6.

Fucile S, Wright P, Chan I, Yee S, Langlais M & Gisel E, 1998, 'Functional Ora–Motor Skills: Do They Change with Age?', *Dysphagia* 13, pp95–201.

Gee P, Palk M & Thatcher C, 1998, 'Nutritional Assessment in Elderly Care – A Team Approach', RCSLT Conference Proceedings, *International Journal of Language and Communication Disorders* 33, supplement.

Giles J & Davison A, 1996, 'SLT and nursing: partners in dysphagia', *RCSLT Bulletin* December, pp10–11.

Gilmour J & Hughes R, 1997, 'Handwashing: still a neglected practice in the clinical area', *British Journal of Nursing* 6 (22), pp1280–84.

Goldstone J, 2000, Personal correspondence from the Director, Centre of Anaesthesia, University College London Medical School.

Greer R, 1998, *Soft Options for Adults who have Difficulty Chewing*, Souvenir Press, UK.

Groher ME, 1984, *Dysphagia: Diagnosis and Management*, Butterworth Heinemann, Boston.

Groher ME, 1990, 'Ethical Dilemmas in Providing Nutrition', *Dysphagia* 5, pp102–9.

Groher ME, 1992, *Dysphagia: Diagnosis and Management*, 2nd edn, Butterworth Heinemann, Boston.

Groher ME & Crary MA, 1997, lecture notes, Dysphagia Conference, May, Cardiff.

Hamdy S & Power M, 1998, 'Cerebral dominance for swallowing', *RCSLT Bulletin,* June, p9.

Hamlet SL, Patterson RL, Fleming SM & Jones LA, 1992, 'Sounds of Swallowing following Total Laryngectomy', *Dysphagia 7,* pp160–65.

Hamlet SL, Nelson RJ & Patterson RL, 1990, 'Interpreting the Sounds of Swallowing: Fluid Flow through the Cricopharyngeus', *Annals of Otology Rhinology and Laryngology 99,* pp749–52.

Haynes S & Hibberd J, 1998, 'Managing tracheostomy and dysphagia', *Speech and Language Therapy in Practice* Autumn, pp8–9.

Health Advisory Service 2000, 1998, *Not Because They are Old,* an independent inquiry into the care of older people on acute wards in general hospitals.

Health Education Authority, 1990, *The Scientific Basis of Dental Health Education. A Policy Document,* 3rd edn, Health Education Authority.

Helm JF, 1989, 'Role of Saliva in Oesophageal Function and Disease', *Dysphagia 4,* pp76–84.

Hendrix TR, 1993, 'Art and Science of History Taking in the Patient with Difficulty Swallowing', *Dysphagia 8,* pp69–73.

Heritage M & Knapp S, 1992, *Nottingham Link Nurse Scheme – Dysphagia Training for Nursing Staff,* Speech and Language Therapy Service, Nottingham Community Health NHS Trust.

Hiiemae K & Palmer J, 1999, 'Food Transport and Bolus Formation During Complete Feeding Sequences on Foods of Different Initial Consistency', *Dysphagia 14,* pp31–42.

Horner J, Braser SR, Massey EW, 1993, 'Aspiration in bilateral stroke patients: a validation study', *Neurology 43,* pp430–33.

Horner J, Massey EW, Riski JE, Lathrop DL & Chase KN, 1988, 'Aspiration Following Stroke: Clinical Correlates and Outcome', *Neurology* 38, pp1359–62.

Horner S, 1999, 'Dysphagia Dilemma: an issue of clinical governance', *RCSLT Bulletin* June, p16.

Hough A, 1997, *Physiotherapy in Respiratory Care*, Stanley Thornes (Publishers), Cheltenham.

Huggins P, Tuomi S & Young C, 1999, 'Effects of Nasogastric Tubes on the Young, Normal Swallowing Mechanism', *Dysphagia* 14, pp157–61.

Hughes H, 1999, 'Silent Aspiration', *Nursing Times* 95 (21).

Hughes TAT & Wiles CM, 1998, 'Neurogenic Dysphagia: the role of the neurologist', *Journal of Neurology Neurosurgery & Psychiatry* 64, pp 569–72.

Johns C, 1993, 'On becoming effective in taking ethical action', *Journal of Clinical Nursing* 2, pp307–12.

Johnson H & Scott A, 1993, *A Practical Approach to Saliva Control*, Communication Skill Builders, Texas.

Jones P, 1998, 'Wind over the desert, wind over the ocean', *RCSLT Bulletin*, May, pp11–12.

Kaplan M & Baum B, 1993, 'The Functions of Saliva', *Dysphagia* 8, pp225–9.

Kahrilas P, 1993, 'Pharyngeal Structure and Function', *Dysphagia* 8, pp303–7.

Kennedy G, 1991, 'A Functional Assessment of Dysphagia', *Speech Therapy in Practice*, April, pp27–8.

Kennedy G, 1992, 'The role of the speech and language therapist in the assessment and management of dysphagia in neurologically impaired patients', *The Fellowship of Postgraduate Medicine* 68, pp545–8.

Kennedy G, Pring T & Fawcus R, 1993, 'No Place for Motor Speech Acts in the Assessment of Dysphagia? Intelligibility and Swallowing Difficulties in Stroke and

Parkinson's Disease Patients', *European Journal of Disorders of Communication* 28, pp213–26.

Klahn M & Perlman A, 1999, 'Temporal and Durational Patterns Associating Respiration and Swallowing', *Dysphagia* 14, pp131–8.

Krawczk K & Codling J, 1998, 'The Dysphagia Audit Project', *RCSLT Conference Proceedings* 33, Supplement.

Langley J, 1988, *Working with Swallowing Disorders*, Speechmark/Winslow Press, Bicester.

Langmore SE, Schatz K & Olsen N, 1988, 'Fibreoptic Endoscopic Examination of Swallowing Safety: A New Procedure', *Dysphagia* 2, pp216–19.

Langmore SE & Logemann JA, 1991, 'After the Clinical Bedside Swallowing Examination: What Next?', *American Journal of Speech and Language Pathology* September, pp13–20.

Langmore S, Terpenning M, Curtis J & Murray J, 1994, 'Risk Factors for Aspiration Pneumonia in the Elderly', short course presented at the ASHA Annual Convention.

Langmore S, Loesche W, Schork T, Terpenning M, Lopatin D & Murray J, 1996, 'Swallowing, Functional and Dental/Oral Status as Predictors of Pneumonia', paper presented at the 5th Annual Dysphagia Research Society Meeting, Aspen, Colorado.

Langmore SE, Terpenning MS, Schork A, Chen Y, Murray J, Lopatin D & Loesche W, 1998, 'Predictors of Aspiration Pneumonia: How Important is Dysphagia?' *Dysphagia* 13, pp69–81.

Langmore S & Murray J, 1999, 'Fibreoptic Endoscopic Evaluation of Swallowing', course notes from study days, held at Charing Cross Hospital, London.

Larsen C, 1998, *HIV-1 and Communication Disorders: What Speech and Hearing Professionals Need to Know*, Singular Publishing Group, San Diego.

Leder S, 1997, 'Videofluoroscopic Evaluation of Aspiration with Visual Examination of the Gag Reflex and Velar Movement', *Dysphagia* 12, pp21–3.

Lennard-Jones JE, 1998, 'Ethical and Legal Aspects of Clinical Hydration and Nutritional Support', British Association for Parenteral and Enteral Nutrition.

Leopold N & Kagel M, 1997, 'Dysphagia – Ingestion or Deglutition? A Proposed Paradigm', *Dysphagia* 12, pp202–6.

Logemann JA, 1993, 'Noninvasive Approaches to Deglutitive Aspiration', *Dysphagia* 8, pp331–3.

Logemann JA, 1998, *Evaluation and Treatment of Swallowing Disorders*, Pro-Ed, Austin, Texas.

Logemann J, Veis S & Colangelo L, 1999, 'A Screening Procedure for Oropharyngeal Dysphagia', *Dysphagia* 14, pp44–51.

Mallet J & Bailey C, 1996, *Manual of Clinical Nursing Procedures,* 4th edn, Blackwell Scientific, Oxford.

Marks L, Fiske J & Hyland K, (2001a), 'Oral Considerations – communication, swallowing, drooling, diet and oral care' Playfer J & Hindle JV (eds), *Parkinson's Disease in the Elderly: A Practical Guide to Assessment and Clinical Management of the Elderly Patient*, Arnold, London.

Marks L, Turner K, O'Sullivan J, Deighton B & Lees A, (2001b), 'Drooling in Parkinson's Disease: A Novel Speeh and Language Therapy Intervention', *International Journal of Language and Communication Disorders* 36 Supplement, pp288–9.

Martin K & Martin J, 1992, 'Meeting the Oral Health Needs of Institutionalised Elderly', *Dysphagia* 7, pp73–80.

Martin B, O'Connor A, Haynes R & McConnel F, 1994, 'Dysphagia Profiles in Patients with Pulmonary Dysfunction: breathing and swallowing interrelationships', short course presented at the ASHA Annual Convention, New Orleans, Louisiana.

Mendelsohn MS, 1994, 'The Modified Barium Swallow Database', *Dysphagia* 9, pp47–53.

Miskovitz P, Weg A & Groher M, 1988, 'Must Dysphagic Patients Always Receive Food and Water?', *Dysphagia* 2, pp125–6.

Mistry B, Samuel L, Bowden S, McArtney R & Roberts D, 1995, 'Simplifying Oral Drug Therapy for Patients with Swallowing Difficulties', *The Pharmaceutical Journal* 254.

Murray J, Langmore S, Ginsberg S & Dostie A, 1996, 'The Significance of Accumulated Oropharyngeal Secretions and Swallowing Frequency in Predicting Aspiration', *Dysphagia* 11, pp99–103.

Nash M, 1988, 'Swallowing Problems in the Tracheostomized Patient', *Otolaryngologic Clinics of North America* 21 (4), pp701–9.

Nathadwarawala KM, McGroary A & Wiles CM, 1994, 'Swallowing in Neurological Outpatients: Use of a Timed Test', *Dysphagia* 9, pp120–9.

Netsell R, 1986, *A Neurological View of Speech Production and the Dysarthrias,* San Diego, College Hill Press.

Nilsson H, Ekberg O, Bulow M & Hindfelt B, 1996, 'Assessment of Respiration in Dysphagic Patients', paper presented at the 5th Annual Dysphagia Research Society Meeting, Aspen, Colorado.

Nilsson H, Ekberg O, Olsson R, Kjellin O & Hindfelt B, 1996, 'Quantitative Assessment of Swallowing in Healthy Adults', *Dysphagia* 11, pp110–16.

Nixon T, 1997, 'Use of Carbonated Liquids in the Treatment of Dysphagia', *A Network Newsletter of Dietetics in Physical Medicine and Rehabilitation.*

O'Loughlin G & Shanley C, 1996, *Swallowing ... on a Plate: A Training Package for Nursing Home Staff Caring for Residents with Swallowing Problems,* Centre for Education and Research on Ageing, Concord.

O'Loughlin G & Shanley C, 1998, 'Swallowing Management in the Nursing Home: A Novel Training Response', *Dysphagia* 13, pp172–83.

Onslow D, 1999, 'Nil by Mouth', *RCSLT Bulletin.*

Palmer JB, Kuhlemeier KV, Tippett DC & Lynch C, 1993, 'A Protocol for the Videofluorographic Swallowing Study', *Dysphagia* 8, pp209–14.

Pannbacker M, Middleton GF & Vekovius GT, 1996, *Ethical Practices in Speech-Language Pathology and Audiology: Case Studies*, Singular Publishing, San Diego.

Perlman AL & Schulze-Delrieu K (eds), 1997, *Deglutition and its Disorders: Anatomy, Physiology, Clinical Diagnosis, and Management*, Singular Publishing, San Diego.

Pulver D, 1999, 'Thickened Drinks: Spit or Swallow', *RCSLT Bulletin* December pp12–13.

Rabeneck L, McCullough LB & Wray NP, 1997, 'Ethically justified, clinically comprehensive guidelines for percutaneous endoscopic gastrostomy tube placement', *The Lancet* 349, pp496–8.

Ravich W, Neumann S, Buchholz D & Jones B, 1998, 'Botulinum Toxin Injection for Pharyngo-Oesophageal Segment (PES) Narrowing in Post-Stroke Dysphagia', abstract of scientific paper presented at the 7th Annual Dysphagia Research Society Meeting, New Orleans, Louisiana.

Reilly S & Carroll L, 1992, 'The use of suction in dysphagic patients: do speech therapists have a role to play?', *CSLT Bulletin* June, p7.

Rice A, 1999, 'Ethical issues around dysphagia', *RCSLT Bulletin* May, p15.

Riches J, 1991, 'In-Service Dysphagia Training Courses for Nurses', *RCSLT Bulletin,* September pp7–8.

Robinson G, Goldstein M & Levine GM, 1987, 'Impact of nutritional status on DRG length of stay', *Journal of Parenteral and Enteral Nutrition* 11, pp49–51.

Rosenbek J, Robbins J, Roecker E, Coyle J & Wood J, 1996, 'A Penetration–Aspiration Scale', *Dysphagia* 11, pp93–8.

Rowland RC, 1988, 'Malpractice in audiology and speech–language pathology', *ASHA* 30 (1), pp45–8.

RCSLT, 1995, 'Collaborative Practice in Dysphagia', The College of Occupational Therapists, The College of Speech and Language Therapists and the Chartered Society of Physiotherapists, London.

RCSLT, 1996, *Communicating Quality 2. Professional Standards for Speech and Language Therapists,* RCSLT London.

RCSLT, 1998a, *Clinical Guidelines by Consensus*, van der Gaag A & Reid D (eds), RCSLT London.

RCSLT, 1998b, 'Legal Pack', Evans P (ed), Legal Resources Group, RCSLT London.

RCSLT, 1999, 'Guidelines I Endoscopic Evaluation of the Vocal Tract, II Tracheo-oesophageal Puncture Prosthesis Procedures, III Radiological Imaging i. Dysphagia ii. The Velopharyngeal Mechanism during Speech Production, for Speech and Language Therapists', RCSLT London.

RCSLT, 2000, *Practice Register and Directory*, RCSLT London.

Sarno MT, 1968, 'Speech Impairment in Parkinson's Disease', *Journal of Neurology, Neurosurgery and Psychiatry* 46, pp140–44.

Schmidt J, Holas M, Halvorsen K & Reding M, 1994, 'Videofluoroscopic Evidence of Aspiration Predicts Pneumonia and Death but not Dehydration following Stroke', *Dysphagia* 9, pp7–11.

Schneiderman LJ, Jecker NS & Jonsen AR, 1990, 'Medical futility: its meaning and ethical implications', *Annals of Internal Medicine* 112, pp949–54.

Scottish Intercollegiate Guidelines Network, 1997, *Management of Patients with Stroke, III: Identification and Management of Dysphagia,* Scottish Intercollegiate Guidelines Network.

Selley WG, Ellis RE, Flack FC, Bayliss CR, Chir B & Pearde VR, 1994, 'The Synchronisation of Respiration and Swallow Sounds with Videofluoroscopy During Swallowing', *Dysphagia* 9, pp162–7.

Selley W, Flack F, Ellis R & Brooks W, 1990, 'The Exeter Dysphagia Assessment Technique', *Dysphagia* 4, pp227–35.

Shaker R, 1993, 'Functional Relationship of the Larynx and Upper GI Tract', *Dysphagia* 8, pp326–30.

Shanahan T, Logemann J, Rademaker A, Pauloski B & Kahrilas P, 1993, 'Chin-Down Posture Effect on Aspiration in Dysphagic Patients', *Arch Phys Med Rehabil* 74.

Sherman B, Nisenboum JM, Jesberger BL, Morrow CA & Jesberger JA, 1999, 'Assessment of Dysphagia with the Use of Pulse Oximetry', *Dysphagia* 14, pp152–6.

Shulman S, 1997, *Information Sheet for Community Pharmacists – Drug Administration to Patients on Enteral Feeds*, Camden and Islington Pharmaceutical Service.

Silverman FH, 1992, 'Legal–ethical considerations, restrictions, and obligations for clinicians who treat communicative disorders', Charles C Thomas, Springfield, IL.

Skipper M, 1997, 'The Cranial Nerves and Muscles Involved in the Process of Swallowing', unpublished.

Slomka J, 1995, 'What Do Apple Pie and Motherhood Have to Do With Feeding Tubes and Caring for the Patient?', *Archives of Internal Medicine* 155, pp1258–63.

Stoschus B & Allescher HD, 1993, 'Drug-Induced Dysphagia', *Dysphagia* 8, pp154–9.

Stroud A, 1999, Cervical auscultation study day lecture notes, St Mary's Hospital, London.

Sugden-Best F, 1999, 'New Ways of Looking at Swallowing – a paradigm shift', *RCSLT Bulletin,* March p15.

Takahashi K, Groher M, Michi K, 1994, 'Methodology for Detecting Swallowing Sounds', *Dysphagia*, Vol 9, pp54–62.

Terpenning M, 1994, 'Oral/Dental and Other Risk Factors in Aspiration Pneumonia', short course presented at the ASHA Annual Convention, New Orleans, Louisiana.

Terry P & Fuller S, 1989, 'Pulmonary Consequences of Aspiration', *Dysphagia* 3, pp179–83.

Torrance A, 1996, 'Off the PEG clinic', *RCSLT Bulletin*, pp10–11.

United Kingdom Central Council for Nursing, Midwifery and Health Visiting, 1997, 'Nurses have responsibility for the feeding of patients', Press release, 8 May 1997.

University College London Hospitals, 1997, 'Infection Control Policy'.

Warland A, 1997, *Physiotherapy Lecture Notes from 'Introductory Course in Eating and Swallowing Difficulties in Adults with Acquired Neurological Disorders'*, Camden and Islington Community Health Services NHS Trust.

Warms T, Champion R & Mortensen L, 1990, *'Paramatta Hospital's Assessment of Dysphagia'*, Adult Speech Pathology Department, Westmead Hospital, New South Wales, Australia.

Webber B & Pryor J, 1995, *Physiotherapy for Respiratory and Cardiac Problems*, Churchill Livingstone, London.

Zenner PM, Losinski DS & Mills RH, 1995, 'Using Cervical Auscultation in the Clinical Dysphagia Examination in Long-Term Care', *Dysphagia* 10, pp27–31.